A HANDBOOK FOR MEDICAL TEACHERS

Fourth Edition

A HANDBOOK FOR MEDICAL TEACHERS
Fourth Edition

DAVID NEWBLE, BSc(Hons), MBChB,
MD, FRACP, DipEd
Professor and Head
Department of Medical Education,
University of Sheffield, UK, and
previously Associate Professor
in Medicine, The University of Adelaide
South Australia

ROBERT CANNON, MA(Hons),
MEdAdmin, DipTertEd
Associate Professor and Director
Advisory Centre for University Education
The University of Adelaide
South Australia

Illustrations by **Zig Kapelis**, MArch, MURP,
DipTCP
Formerly Senior Lecturer in Architecture
The University of Adelaide, South Australia

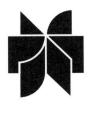

KLUWER ACADEMIC PUBLISHERS
DORDRECHT / BOSTON / LONDON

Published by Kluwer Academic Publishers, PO Box 17, 3300 AA
Dordrecht, The Netherlands

Sold and distributed in North, Central and South America by Kluwer
Academic Publishers, 101 Philip Drive, Norwell, MA 02018, USA

In all other countries. sold and distributed by Kluwer Academic
Publishers, Distribution Center, PO Box 322, 3300 AH Dordrecht, The
Netherlands

ISBN 0-7923-7092-9

A catalogue record for this book is available from the Library of
Congress

Printed on acid-free paper

Fourth edition © 2001 David Newble and Robert Cannon

First edition published 1983 as *A Handbook for Clinical Teachers*
Reprinted 1984, 1985
Second edition published 1987
Reprinted 1990
Third edition published 1994
Reprinted 1996

Printed and bound in Great Britain by MPG Books Limited, Bodmin,
Cornwall

CONTENTS

PREFACE

The first edition of this book was published in 1983 as a response to a concern that few resources were available to the medical teacher wishing to gain a perspective on basic educational principles and their application to teaching. Its success led to revised editions published in 1987 and 1994. We have also been delighted to find the book in use in many countries and there are now several non-English versions.

Over these years the climate for educational reform has improved considerably. Higher education institutions are responding to both internal and external pressures to improve the quality of their courses and the teaching performance of individual staff members. Institutions are encouraging educational innovation, tackling the problem of rewards and promotion for contributions to teaching, supporting staff development activities, and introducing staff appraisal and quality assurance procedures. Thus, the need of individual teachers for practical help in meeting these changing expectations is becoming increasingly evident.

Preparing this fourth edition has presented us with numerous challenges. Clearly much has changed even since 1994. For example the rapid growth in the use of the Internet and other teaching technologies raises many questions. The pressures on institutions to cut costs and to teach 'more efficiently' has intensified a move towards greater accountability. Participation in some form of 'teach the teachers how to teach' programme is increasingly becoming mandatory and in some countries may even become an external requirement to be in charge of university courses. We know our book has been used successfully as a basic text for such programmes.

In keeping with these changes we have updated all chapters and have attempted to cover recent developments we feel have general application. In doing so we have remained mindful of the original design of the book to be easy to read and to focus on the practical needs of the medical teacher. It is not our intent that this be a comprehensive text on medical education. However, we have continued to provide key references and guided reading for each chapter and an appendix which lists some of the more widely read journals and major international meetings on medical education.

We have, as usual, planned this book so that you can go directly to the topic of immediate interest. However, with this edition we have commenced with an overview of the considerable research that has been forthcoming in the last 20 years on how students learn and the importance of this for the teacher. It puts up front an emphasis on the many factors which influence the effectiveness of our activities as teachers. If we are not aware of these, and do not take them into account, then much of what we do may be undermined.

Finally we would like to express our appreciation to the staff at Kluwer Academic Publishers for their continued support. The help of our secretary Carol Icke is specifically acknowledged and appreciated.

David Newble
Robert Cannon

1: HELPING STUDENTS LEARN

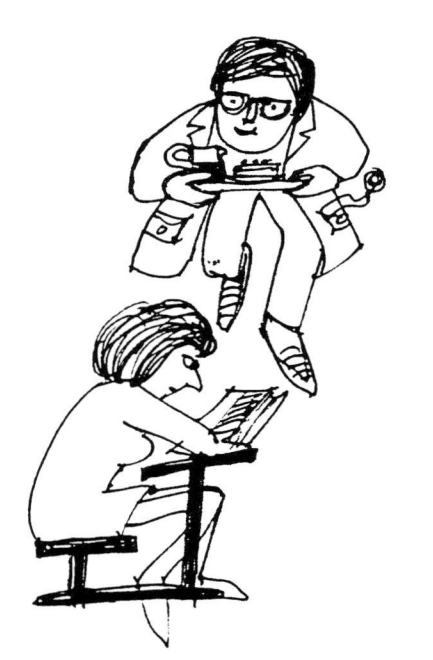

INTRODUCTION

If you inspected a copy of the previous edition of our book you would notice that this chapter had moved from being the last to the first. While this book is intended to be very practical in its approach we believe there are important reasons for the early introduction of rather more theoretical perspectives. The first is that research and thinking about learning is yielding insights into teaching which helps us construct practical advice on a firmer foundation than previously. The second reason is because of the fundamental challenge it provides to the more traditional views and stereotypes that prevail about students and learning in higher education.

Teachers have been primarily interested in what and how much students learn and elaborate assessment methods have been devised to measure these. But in the last quarter of the twentieth century a considerable body of evidence accumulated which suggested that we need to become much more concerned with how our students learn and the contextual forces that shape their learning. We need to appreciate that some of our students are having difficulties with their studies arising not just from their lack of application or psychosocial problems, but from specific ways in which they study and learn. We must also appreciate that many of their difficulties are directly attributable to the assumptions we make about them, and the way we teach, organize courses, and conduct assessments.

HOW STUDENTS LEARN

Although there has been an enormous amount of research into learning over very many years, no one has yet come up with a coherent set of principles that would adequately predict or explain how students learn in any particular context. There have been psychological studies, studies in the neurosciences, in cognitive science, evolutionary studies, anthropological studies, and even archaeological evidence about learning to name a few! The paper by Marchese, available from the Web, provides a fascinating, scholarly and entertaining introduction to all this intellectual effort.

It was not until 1976 that a landmark study by two Swedish researchers, Marton and Saljo, shifted the traditional research focus from teachers and teaching onto what students actually think and do in real situations. They reported that all students have distinctive **approaches to learning** that we now understand are influenced by many factors, as shown in Figure 1.1. The chain of events in learning and the links between them are the focus of much current research effort and so are likely to be further refined over time. We attempt to summarise current understanding here.

FIGURE 1.1.
A MODEL OF STUDENT LEARNING

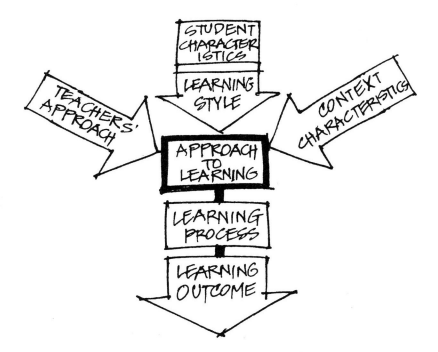

One of the factors influencing learning is **student characteristics** and these include individual differences, students' previous learning experiences and current understanding of the subject. Other influences can be grouped under **context characteristics**. These include, especially, the ethos of the department organizing the course and the characteristics of the curriculum. Closely related to this is the **teachers' approach** to teaching (a characteristic we discuss in more detail below).

The effect of these factors is to influence **students' perceptions** of their context and the **learning approach** that is expected of them. Students can be observed to use one of three broad approaches to learning, commonly called surface, deep and strategic.

Students adopting a **surface approach** to learning are predominantly motivated by a concern to complete the course or by a fear of failure. In fact, the emotional aspects of students' perceptions of their context is beginning to receive attention and it is emerging that anxiety, fear of failure and low self-esteem are associated with surface approaches. Surface approach students intend to fulfil the assessment requirements of the course by using **learning processes** such as acquiring information, mechanical memorisation without understanding it, and reproducing it on demand in a test. The focus is on the material or task and not on its meaning or purpose. The **learning outcome** is, at best, a memorisation of factual information and perhaps a superficial level of understanding.

In contrast, students adopting a **deep approach** are motivated by an interest in the subject matter and a need to make sense of things and to interpret knowledge. Their intention is to reach an understanding of the material. The process of achieving this varies between individual students and between students in different academic disciplines. The operation learner relies on a logical step-by-step approach with a cautious acceptance of generalisations only when based on evidence. There is an appropriate attention to factual and procedural detail which may include memorisation for understanding. This process is most prevalent in science departments. On the other hand, the comprehension learner uses a process in which the initial concern is for the broad outlines of ideas and their interconnections with previous knowledge. Such students make use of analogies and attempt to give the material personal meaning. This process is more evident in arts and social science departments. However, another process is that used by the so-called versatile learner for whom the outcome is a deep level of understanding based on a knowledge of broad principles supported by a sound factual basis. Versatile learning does not preclude the use of memorisation when the need arises, as it frequently does in science-based courses, but the students do so with a totally different intent from those using the surface approach.

Students demonstrating the **strategic approach** to learning may be seen to use processes similar to both the deep and surface learner. The fundamental difference lies in their

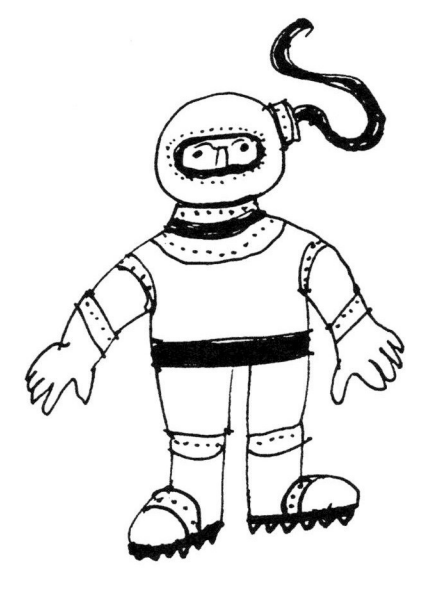

motivation and intention. Such students are motivated by the need to achieve high marks and to compete with others. The outcome is a variable level of understanding that depends on what is required by the course and, particularly, the assessments.

The **learning outcomes** can be broadly described in terms of quantity and quality of learning. The outcomes we would hope from a university or college education are very much those resulting from the deep approach. Disturbingly, the evidence we have suggests that these outcomes may not always be encouraged or achieved by students. Indeed, as we stress repeatedly, there is good reason to believe that many of our teaching approaches, curriculum structures and, particularly, our assessment methods, may be inhibiting the use of the deep approach and supporting and rewarding the use of surface or strategic approaches to learning. This appears to be particularly so for medical students undertaking traditional curricula (see article by Newble and Entwistle).

NON-TRADITIONAL STUDENTS AND THEIR LEARNING

Medical schools now enrol significant numbers of students who do not come directly from high school. Students from overseas and older students entering without the usual prerequisites are just two examples of what we might call 'non-traditional students' in medical education.

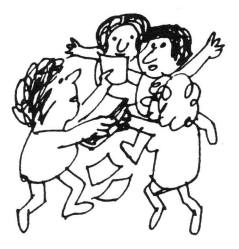

There has been something of an explosion in the research and writing about such students and their learning. This literature is very revealing. In broad terms, it is showing us that any so-called 'problems' with these students are often the result of ill-informed attitudes and educational practices, in short, a result of poor teaching. This confirms the importance of creating a positive learning environment rather than seeking fault with students.

Students from different cultural backgrounds

One thing we are sure you will have noticed in your institution or from your reading is that stereotypes are attached to students from different cultural backgrounds. One of these stereotypes is that students, particularly those from Asia, are rote learners. Yet many studies have shown that these students score at least as well and sometimes higher than western students on measures of deep learning. You may also have noticed how there seems to be a disproportionate number of these Asian students who receive academic distinctions and prizes!

This apparent 'paradox' – adopting surface approaches such as rote learning but demonstrating high achievement in academic courses – has been the subject of much investigation. What is emerging is that researchers have assumed that memorisation was equated with mechanical rote learning. But memorisation is not a simple concept. It is intertwined with understanding such as when you might rote learn a poem to assist in the processes of interpretation and understanding. Thus the traditional Confucian heritage way of memorisation can have different purposes. Sometimes it can be for mechanical rote learning. But it is also used to deepen and develop understanding. The paradox of these learners is solved when memorisation is seen as an important part of the process leading to understanding.

We encourage you to read further about these issues, and about some of the other problematic cultural stereotypes (such as Asian student participation in classes) in the Guided Reading sources listed at the end of the chapter. They will not only help you to assist these students become more effective learners but also provide a clearer understanding about the processes of learning more generally.

Older students

The literature in this area also makes interesting reading. It tells us is that older students are generally little different from the more traditional entry younger students, and sometimes better in important ways. Figure 1.2 summarises some of the key findings presented in Hartley's book.

USING NEW TECHNOLOGY AND LEARNING

The literature in this field tends to be of two main kinds: that which has researched the impact of technologies such as computers on learning processes and outcomes, and the

FIGURE 1.2.
OLDER AND YOUNGER STUDENTS
(AFTER HARTLEY)

When compared with younger students, mature students:

- usually perform as well academically, and sometimes better;
- score better on measures of deep learning and time management;
- are generally similar on measures of ability;
- are no different in preference for instructional styles or in conceptions of what constitutes good teaching.

more general and speculative literature. Given the vast span of this literature over issues and time, and given the different methods used by researchers, it is difficult to draw too many useful generalisations to help you in your teaching other than:

- research on the impact of technologies such as computer-aided learning shows small but nevertheless positive effects on learning and attitudes;
- studies of the impact of specific technologies (such as video and electronic mail) on learning shows a great diversity of outcomes which reflect both the nature and potential capability of the technology and, importantly, the way it is used by teachers and learners;
- the general literature is pointing to ways in which technology, sensitively used, can contribute to a range of improved learning processes and to outcomes such as enhanced tools for learning; improved flexibility for those with access to the technology; individualising learning; and more student activity.

If you are hoping to find spectacular learning outcomes from using the new technologies you may be disappointed at this stage. Equally we believe there are opportunities to address many of the ills of education by using modern technology to support quality learning.

LEARNING MORE EFFECTIVELY

The concepts outlined above are not only supported by a growing body of research evidence, but also match the kinds of things good teachers know and do when teaching their students. We are now in a better position than we were in earlier editions of this book to make suggestions

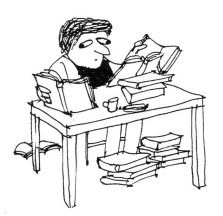

and offer practical advice based on the accumulating research evidence and the experiences of practicing teachers in higher education.

Improving the learning environment

This must be considered at various levels. At the broadest level is the educational philosophy underlying the whole curriculum. There may be little you can do about this, but there is evidence that students from schools using traditional teaching practices are more likely to adopt surface approaches to a greater degree than students from programmes that are more student-centred. You may be able to gauge where the educational philosophy of your own discipline or curriculum fits and predict the likely effect it has on your students' approach to learning.

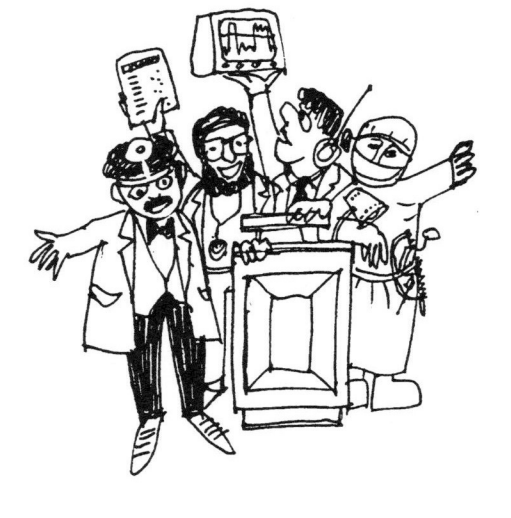

At another level, and one where you might be able to exert some influence, is the structuring of the curriculum. You should be aware that the fragmentation of the curriculum into a large number of courses or course components taught by different teachers may be counter-productive to the development of deep approaches. The time available to each is limited and so the opportunities for students to come to grips with the deeper implications and perspectives of subject matter are similarly restricted. Such fragmentation has become increasingly apparent in medical curricula.

In recent years many different teaching methods have been re-discovered or developed not from research studies but from the practice and the experience of thoughtful teachers. Perhaps the one which has made the greatest impact is problem-based learning which is discussed in detail in Chapter 7.

There are other methods and approaches which are more student-centred and appear more likely to encourage deep learning and enhance learning outcomes. Some of the principles which these incorporate are shown in Figure 1.3. They may be reflected in activities such as research projects, peer teaching, case-based learning, learning portfolios and so on. In general, this means that the primary focus of the teacher should be to provide a learning environment which is stimulating, based on interaction, and which emphasizes the responsibility of the student to participate actively in learning activities.

Students are more likely to adopt a deeper approach to their learning and achieve quality learning outcomes when teachers provide for:

● intrinsic motivation and curiosity
● student independence
● student choice
● opportunities to work with other people
● an environment that is challenging, supportive and low threat
● frequent, constructive and useable feedback
● well-structured and clear organisation
● active involvement in realistic learning tasks
● an emphasis on higher-level objectives
● practice and reinforcement

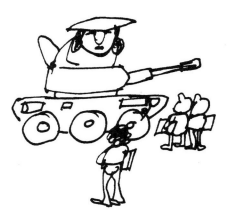

The major differences between student-centred learning and conventional teaching are listed in Figure 1.4.

As most teachers reading this book will be working in a conventional institution, it is important to introduce into courses those measures which might encourage the use of the deep approach. Some other measures you can implement are listed below:

● Ensure that the course objectives specify more than just facts and technical skills by giving suitable emphasis to higher-level intellectual skills, such as problem-solving and critical thinking; to working collaboratively with others; and to the exploration and development of appropriate attitudes.
● Introduce teaching activities which require students to demonstrate a deep understanding of the subject matter. Do not allow students to 'get away' with only reproducing factual information and take a genuine interest in what they say and do as indicators of their learning.
● Reduce the time allocated to didactic teaching to allow more time for students to work with other people and for self-directed learning.
● Decrease the amount of factual material that has to be memorised. Both pressure of time and overloading with content is known to encourage the surface approach even in those intending to use the deep

Student-centred learning

- students have responsible and active role (in planning their learning, interacting with teachers and other students, researching, assessing)
- students required to make choices about what and how to learn
- emphasis on integrating learning across the curriculum
- emphasis on enquiry-type activities
- teacher as guide, mentor and facilitator of learning
- intrinsic motivation (interest, curiosity, responsibility)
- focus on cooperative learning
- learning can occur anywhere
- greater flexibility in learning and teaching
- greater flexibility in assessment with self and peer assessment becoming more common
- long-term perspective: emphasis on lifelong learning

Conventional teaching

- students often passive (no role in planning learning, sitting in lectures)
- most decisions are made by the teacher
- emphasis on learning this subject only
- emphasis on receiving information
- teacher as expert dispenser of knowledge and controller of activities
- extrinsic motivation (grades, teacher praise)
- individual learning and competition between students
- learning confined to fixed teaching venues (lecture rooms, libraries, labs.)
- relatively inflexible arrangements
- assessment seen as the responsibility of the teacher with examinations as an important focus
- short-term perspective: emphasis on completing assigned work and learning for the examination

approach. These problems are prevalent in many science-based medical courses.

- Spend more contact time in helping students to understand and use basic principles and in understanding the difficulties they may be having. Get into the habit of expecting students to explain answers to questions. The frequent use of the word 'why' will quickly establish if the answer is based on memorisation or on an understanding of an underlying principle.
- Evaluate the extent to which students find you or their context threatening and take measures to eliminate or reduce this as much as you can, taking care to maintain acceptable levels of intellectual challenge.
- Most importantly, review the assessment procedures. This is a critical task. If the assessment, course content and learning methods do not match the course

objectives, then one could be the world's greatest teacher and make little impact on the students' learning. For example, an over-reliance on objective tests of low level recall (true-false, multiple choice) will almost certainly encourage the use of surface strategies. If you aim to have students understand the subject, then you must introduce forms of assessment which require them to demonstrate this understanding. This may mean the re-introduction of essays, and the use of research projects, self and peer assessment, and so on.

Modifying teaching approaches

Evidence is being found that there is a relationship between a **teacher's approach** to teaching and the quality of student learning outcomes. Research and thinking about teaching over nearly thirty years shows that teachers hold rather different 'theories' of teaching and learning which influence their approach to teaching. Very broadly, there are teachers who believe their job is to cover the subject systematically by transmitting content to students. Failure to learn the content is seen to be the fault of the student. It appears that teachers who have this approach are more likely to encourage surface learning among their students.

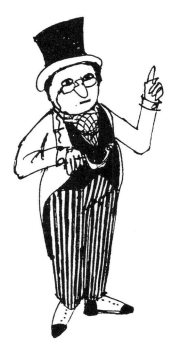

On the other hand there are teachers who consider their main role is to assist students' understanding and conceptual change. They focus on what the students do and what learning outcomes result from their activity. Failure to learn is considered to be just as likely to be due to some failure in the way in which the curriculum was planned and implemented, as it is to be a deficit in students or their teachers. Such teachers, who would describe their teaching as student-focused, are less likely to encourage surface learning approaches among their students. We strongly suggest you read the article by Trigwell, Prosser and Waterhouse to deepen your understanding of these important relationships.

The bottom line is that teachers need to be aware of their approach and the impact this may have on the **learning approach** of their students. We are not in a position to modify your beliefs and theories here, although we hope that some of this information may help! However we can suggest you experiment with several of the student-centred strategies described in this book if you wish to encourage high quality student learning.

Improving learning skills

There seems little doubt that good learning and study skills contribute to improved academic performance, though in themselves they are not a guarantee of success. Equally, possessing learning skills is now seen as having a lifelong relevance and not just limited to good grades in an end-of-course examination.

These lifelong learning skills can be developed in your courses and include self-organising skills; skill in deeper learning strategies such as analysis, judgement, synthesis and application; locating, retrieving, interpreting, evaluating and managing information; and the skills of breadth and depth of vision and the capacity to appreciate the interrelated nature of knowledge.

It is clear that some students continue to use study skills and approaches which are inappropriate and ineffective. It is important for teachers to identify such students as they may need help with specific study skill counselling. Many of these students become persistent poor performers and it can be very rewarding for both teacher and students to realise that a specific remedy is available.

For further information and help with specific study skill counselling we suggest you look at some of the guides and manuals that are now available. It might also be helpful to consult the student counselling service or teaching support unit at your institution.

GUIDED READING

A very good general text on learning is *Learning and Studying, A Research Perspective* by J. Hartley, Routledge, London, 1998. This is a particularly helpful reference for teachers as it simply and comprehensively discusses learning from a range of different research perspectives and makes practical suggestions on ways in which teachers can improve learning for their students. It contains sections that review the literature on older students and technologies discussed above.

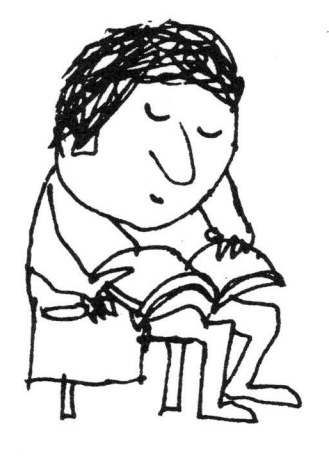

Other useful texts covering the approaches to learning literature are *The Experience of Learning* (2nd edition) by F. Marton, D. Hounsell and N. Entwistle (eds), Scottish Academic Press, Edinburgh, 1997 and *Teaching for Quality Learning at University* by J. Biggs, Buckingham, Open University Press, 1999.

For an introduction to practical strategies and theoretical issues in lifelong learning we recommend C. Knapper and A. Cropley, *Lifelong Learning in Higher Education* (2nd edition) Kogan Page, London, 2000, and P. Candy, G. Crebert and J. O'Leary, *Developing Lifelong Learning Through Undergraduate Education*, Australian Government Publishing Service, Canberra, 1994. Both contain many exemplars of lifelong learning practices in higher education.

Recent editions, from around 1997, of the journal *Higher Education Research and Development* have included several helpful papers about Asian students. A particularly relevant edition is Volume 16, Number 1, April 1997: 'Common misconceptions about students from South-East Asia studying in Australia' by D. Chalmers and S. Volet.

A very useful book containing detailed advice on how to study is *A Guide to Learning Independently* by L. Marshall and F. Rowland, Open University Press, UK, 1999. Though written for students it is a valuable resource for teachers.

Books and articles referred to in this chapter:

F. Marton and R. Saljo (1976). On qualitative differences in learning: I. Outcomes and process. *British Journal of Educational Psychology*, **46**: 4-11.

K. Trigwell, M. Prosser, and F. Waterhouse (1999). Relations between teachers' approaches to teaching and students' approaches to learning. *Higher Education*, **37**: 57-70.

T. Marchese. *The Adult Learner in Higher Education and the Workplace; The New Conversations about Learning*. Available:
http://www.newhorizons.org/lrnbus_marchese.html

D. Newble and N. Entwistle (1988). Learning styles and approaches: implications for medical education. *Medical Education*, **20**, 162-175.

2: TEACHING IN LARGE GROUPS

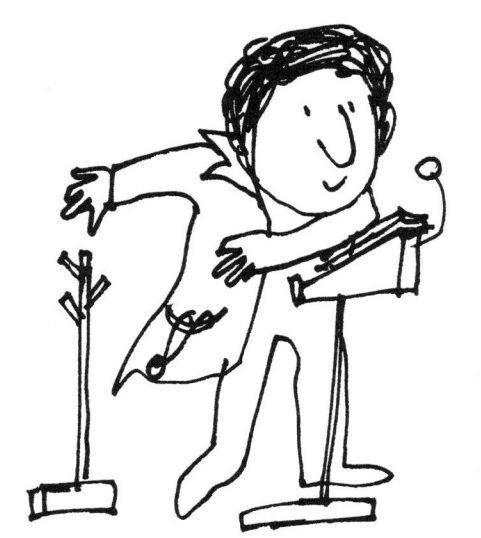

INTRODUCTION

Large group teaching is often thought of as the same as lecturing. While the lecture is still a very common teaching method in most medical schools we want to encourage you to think more creatively about how you might best use your time when faced with a large group of students. There are good educational reasons for moving away from the traditional approach of 'lecturing' to groups of passive students to strategies which introduce more active learning. While the solution to this concern may, in part, involve replacing the notion of large group teaching with alternative approaches, such as small group teaching or distance learning, we recognize that other factors may preclude such options. Should this be the case we believe that you can employ a range of techniques in the large group situation which will engage your students enthusiastically in active learning, provide them with immediate feedback and build a productive and scholarly relationship.

Why do we want to support you in this move towards putting students at the centre of your thinking? Because the evidence continues to mount that, although the lecture is as effective as other methods to transmit information (but not more effective), it is not as effective as other methods to stimulate thinking, to inspire interest in a subject, to teach behavioural skills, or to change attitudes. These are among the objectives that many medical teachers aspire to when they lecture. On the other hand, if we seriously wish to foster lifelong learning skills and attitudes among our students, one of the worst things we can do is to encourage and reward the kinds of passivity that the lecture method commonly provides.

This chapter seeks to provide you with practical suggestion on how you might approach the task if asked to give a 'lecture'.

THE CONTEXT OF LARGE GROUP TEACHING

An important preliminary step in your preparation is to find out as much as you can about the context of your teaching in the overall teaching programme or course. Unfortunately this context is often ill defined and may be only a title in a long list of topics given out by the department or school. However, do try to find out as much as you can. This means enquiring about such things as:

- what students have been taught (and what they may know),
- what the purpose of your teaching session is to be,
- what resources, such as library materials, are available for students,
- what the assessment arrangements for the course or unit are,
- what methods have been used to teach students in the past.

This last point is most important. You may wish, after reading this chapter, to try out some new ideas with students. Beware! Students do appreciate good teaching but may resent the use of some techniques that seem irrelevant to their purposes, to the course aims, and to the way their learning is assessed. When introducing new learning and teaching techniques you must carefully explain the purpose of them to students. Be prepared for some resistance, especially from senior students if they do not appreciate the connection between the techniques and the assessment arrangements.

The course co-ordinator, curriculum committee, head of department and other teachers in the course are all potential sources of advice and assistance to you. However, do not be surprised if you are told that you are the expert and that it is your responsibility to know what students should be taught! If this happens you should insist on some help to review what happened in the past. To do otherwise is to teach in an academic vacuum.

WHAT ABOUT NON-TRADITIONAL STUDENTS?

A declining proportion of university students enter directly from local secondary schools. Given the growing numbers of non-traditional students, such as international students from different cultural and linguistic backgrounds and mature-age students, it is important that you note the composition of your class and consider this in your planning. What can be done? An essential starting point is to base your teaching on sound educational principles which are likely to be beneficial for *all* students in your class.

In addition, however, you can assist your students from diverse backgrounds by instituting practices that provide modelling, resources for increased comprehension, and enhanced opportunities for social contact.

Modelling the kinds of learning objectives you have will be important for all students including those who come from cultures where the traditional authority of teachers and authors is strongly valued and not to be questioned. For example, plan to model critical or analytical thinking by publicly questioning a set text and explicitly demonstrating through your own thinking approaches the ways in which scholars in your discipline test the validity of claims made.

Resources for increased comprehension will be welcomed by the majority of your class, but particularly those students for whom the language of instruction is not their first language, and for hearing and sight-impaired students, among others. What can you do? A short list would include: presenting an overview and structure to each session; using concrete examples of the principles you are teaching; linking one session to the next and to the one preceding it; providing clear, large, legible over-heads or slides, handouts, outlines of the teaching session; audio taping of classes and the maintenance of a tape library; posting class notes on the Internet or an intranet; and indicating supporting references in books and journals and stating why each reference is important or how it relates to the topic.

Using technology in teaching large groups can also be a valid strategy to address some of these issues. See below for ideas on how you might proceed with this.

Social contact will be achieved in large group teaching when you use some of the group-based approaches described here. One of the most under-used resources in higher education is the students themselves, so plan ways in which you might constructively use the experience and knowledge of particular students or groups of students in your teaching. Not only will the learning be enriched but an opportunity for some social contact between yourself and the students will have been provided.

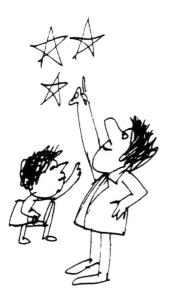

PREPARING FOR LARGE GROUP TEACHING

What is the purpose of your teaching?

Having clarified the context of your large group teaching session you need to ask yourself 'What is its purpose?' This is a question you should always ask so that you have a clear idea about matching ends with means.

A possible range of answers is given below, many of which will overlap.

- To **encourage** thinking skills.
  Examples: Interpret a set of statistical data; evaluate a research proposal; criticize a journal article or medical treatment plan; apply earlier learning to a novel situation.
- To **construct** an academic argument.
  Example: Present the pro and con arguments with respect to a health policy issue.
- To **present** students with information about a subject.
  Example: Review and comment on the research on a particular subject.
- To **demonstrate** a procedure, a way of thinking, or approach to problem solving.
  Examples: Lead students through a line of reasoning about a problem; demonstrate a clinical or technical procedure.

Resolving the purpose of your large group teaching will be a useful benchmark throughout the process of preparation, presentation and final evaluation.

Having clarified the context and purpose to the best of your ability the time has come to get down to some detailed planning. The best way to start is to write down the outcomes you hope to achieve in your teaching session(s). We say 'write down' advisedly because nothing clarifies the mind more than putting pen to paper!

Identify the content

Now set about identifying the content. We suggest you start by initially jotting down the main ideas, theories and examples that come to mind regarding the central purpose of your teaching session. This should be done spontaneously, without any particular concern for the order in which you may eventually wish to organise your material. Figure 2.1 illustrates a way of doing this that has been found to be helpful by staff attending our courses for new academic staff.

FIGURE 2.1.
METHOD OF IDENTIFYING THE
CONTENT FOR A LECTURE

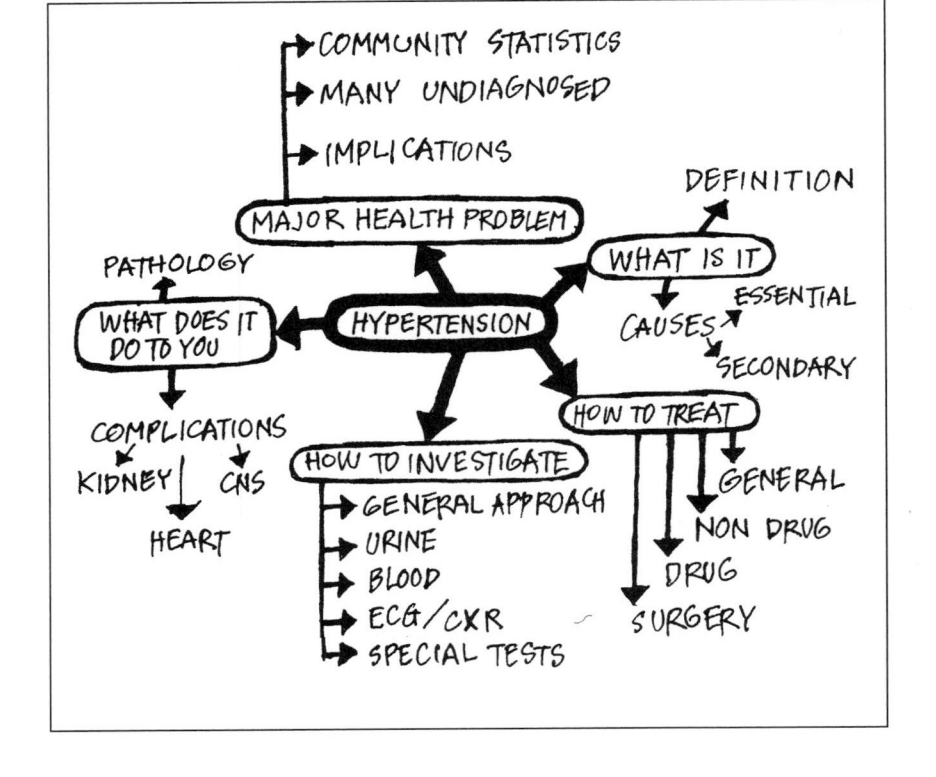

The topic (in the example, taken from a medical lecture on hypertension) is placed in the centre of the paper and the main points to be made are written down as indicated. When the main ideas are identified, further points will tend to branch out as you think more carefully about them. This process is continued until you have exhausted all your ideas. You may at this stage discover that you need to read around some of the ideas in order to refine them or to bring yourself up to date.

During this exercise you will find that illustrative examples of key points come to mind. Jot these down also. In addition you should be on the look out for illustrations from which you might prepare audiovisual aids and teaching materials. Appropriate jokes or cartoons may be collected during this exercise. And, most importantly, make a note of short activities or exercises that you can use as a basis for student activity.

Finalise the plan

Now you must finalise your teaching plan. The rough content plan must be transformed into a structure, which follows some kind of logical sequence. There is no single best way of doing so but you may prefer a formal structure from which to work. The important point is to have a structure and make this clear to students when you are teaching.

One such structure is seen in Figure 2.2.

FIGURE 2.2.
LARGE GROUP TEACHING PLAN

1 Introduction and overview
    a. Describe the purpose of the session
    b. Outline the key areas to be covered

2 First key point
    a. Development of ideas
    b. Use of examples
    c. Restatement of first key point
    d. Task/exercise/question for students

3 Second key point
    a. Development of ideas
    b. Use of examples
    c. Restatement of first and second points
    d. Task/exercise/question for students

4 Third key point
    a. Development of ideas
    b. Use of examples
    c. Restatement of first, second and third points
    d. Task/exercise/question for students

5 Summary and conclusion

This is the classical **content-oriented plan**. We hope you may wish to be more ambitious and use other plans which have the potential to more effectively demonstrate how knowledge is discovered and organised in your discipline. These plans require extra thought but done well are likely to be rewarding to both you and your students.

An example of such an alternative is the **problem-focused plan**. It can be structured as follows:

- Introduction: Presentation of the problem (e.g. as a case)
- First possible solution
- Second possible solution
- Third possible solution etc
- Comparison and appropriateness of possible solutions
- Summary and Conclusions

Another adaptation is the **academic-argument plan**. The order in which you place arguments in this structure appears to be critical. The order suggested is:

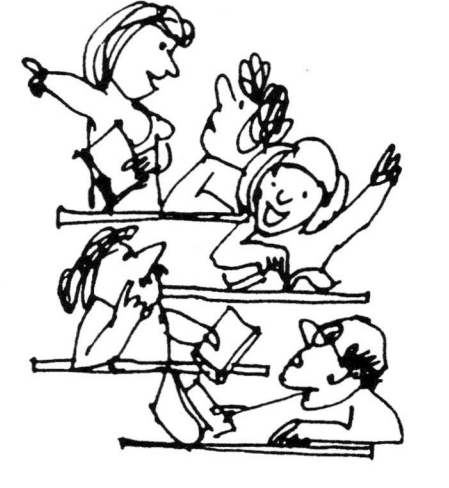

- Introduction: Overview of teacher's position and supporting arguments
- First major point: Presentation of counter-arguments
- Second major point: Discussion/refutation of counter-arguments
- Third major point: Arguments in favour of teacher's position
- Conclusion: Restatement of teacher's position

These examples imply that all large group sessions are complete in themselves. In reality, of course, this may not be the situation. Most will be part of a series on a particular topic or theme. Consequently, they will need to be linked together to provide continuity from one session to the next. In other words, you will need to modify the plans suggested above to suit the demands of your teaching as it proceeds through the series.

The plans illustrate the general question you will have to answer as you organize your material: 'How will I sequence the ideas I wish to present?' Sometimes the sequence might be indicated by the nature of the material to be presented. However, apparently logical sequences may not always be optimal for student learning and you should give some thought to the ways in which student interests, their knowledge and approaches to learning suggest sequences of presentation. Some possible sequences are:

- Proceed from observations of reality, such as a brief in-class activity (e.g. a case study, an exercise or short test, a short film or video, a Classroom Assessment Technique [see below], or a demonstration), to abstract ideas, theories and principles. This is sometimes called an inductive approach to teaching.

- Proceed from generalisations to particular examples and applications. This is a deductive approach – a reversal of the inductive sequence outlined above.
- Proceed from simple ideas and applications to more complex ones.
- Proceed from what students can be expected to know to what students do not know.
- Proceed from common misconceptions to explanation and clarification.
- Proceed from a whole view to a more detailed view.

PRESENTING THE LARGE GROUP TEACHING SESSION

Having decided what you intend to teach, you must now give careful attention to how you are going to present it to the students. Let us assume that it is to be your first contact with this group of students. You may wish to obtain their attention initially by devising an arresting opening. Ways of doing this are limited only by your personality and your imagination. An appropriate anecdote, a video clip, a quotation or a discussion with a few of the group may generate interest.

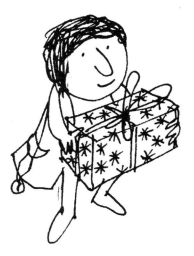

However, it must be borne in mind that the attention of the students ought to be engaged by the material rather than the personality of the teacher. The danger of the latter has become known as the 'Dr Fox effect' based on an experiment where an actor (Dr Fox) gave a lecture comprising meaningless double-talk which fooled experienced listeners into believing that they had participated in a worthwhile and stimulating learning experience.

Starting the session

Particular attention needs to be given to the way you begin. For many teachers, this is the most difficult aspect of teaching a large group. It is essential to decide beforehand exactly how you intend to start. Do not leave this decision until you are facing the students. Perhaps the easiest way to start is to explain the purpose of the teaching session and how it is organized. An outline on the board or on a transparency showing your teaching plan is a good way of doing this. Such visual material will take attention away from yourself, give you something to talk to and allow you to settle down. Writing the plan on the board gives students a permanent reminder of the structure of your session.

Once you become more confident, other issues should be considered. It is good practice to arrive early and chat with some of the students to establish their level of previous knowledge. Alternatively, you can start by asking a few pertinent questions, taking care that this is done in a non-threatening manner. Should you establish that serious deficiencies in knowledge are present you must be flexible enough to try and correct them rather than continue on regardless.

Varying the format

You should now give attention to the body of the large group session. Student attention must be considered. A purely verbal presentation will be ineffective and will contribute to a fall-off in the level of attention. You should therefore be planning ways of incorporating some of the techniques described in the next section. Figure 2.3. shows us that levels of attention and learning will fall progressively. No more than 20 minutes should go by before the students are given a learning activity or before the teaching technique is significantly altered. Ways of doing this include posing questions or testing the students, generating discussion among students and using an audiovisual aid. These active learning strategies are discussed in more detail later.

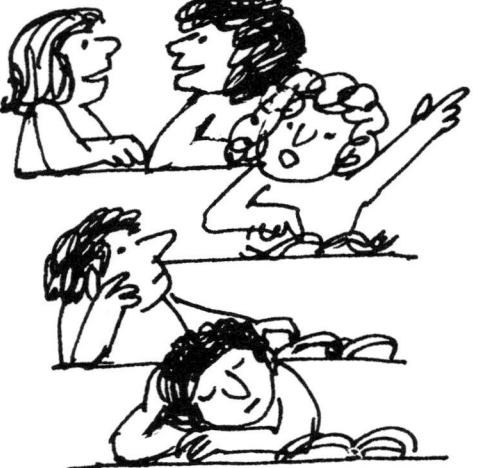

FIGURE 2.3.
HYPOTHESIZED PATTERN OF STUDENT LEVEL OF PERFORMANCE SHOWING A PROGRESSIVE FALL IN ATTENTION AND LEARNING DURING AN UNINTERRUPTED LECTURE AND CONTRASTING THIS WITH THE GAIN OBTAINED FROM INTRODUCING A REST PERIOD (AFTER BLIGH)

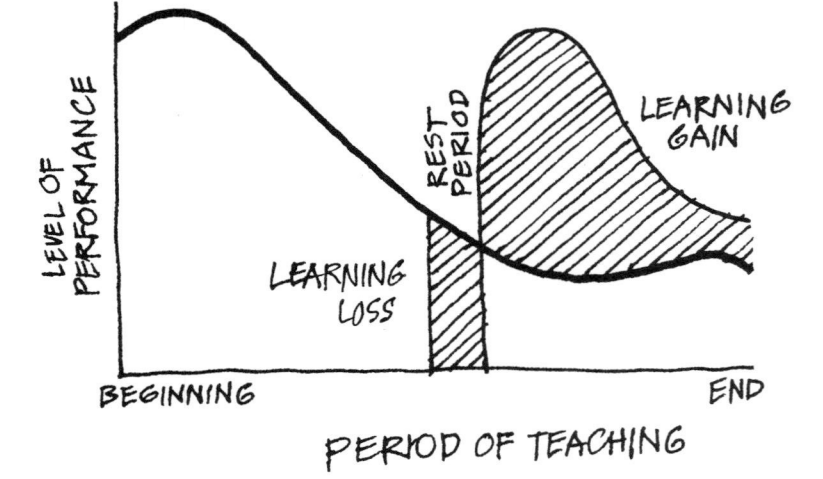

Finishing the session

The conclusion is as important as the introduction. Your closing comments should also be well prepared. The last things that you say are the ones the students are most likely to remember. This will be the opportunity to reiterate the key points you hope to have made. You may also wish to direct students to additional reading at this time, but be reasonable in your expectations and give them a clear indication of what is essential and why it is essential as opposed to what you think is merely desirable. A couple of minutes near the conclusion to allow them to consolidate and read their notes is a worthwhile technique to use from time to time.

Rehearsal and check

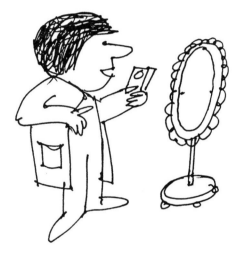

Some of the best teachers we know find it very helpful to rehearse or to try-out some parts of their teaching so this may be even more important for the less experienced. However, the purpose of the rehearsal should not be to become word perfect, and it is impossible to rehearse the outcomes of activities you give your students. A rehearsal will often reveal that you are attempting to cram too much into the time and that some of your visual aids are poorly prepared or difficult to see from the rear of the theatre. The value of a rehearsal will be much enhanced if you invite along a colleague to act as the audience and to provide critical comments and to help you check out projectors, seating, lighting, air conditioning, and other physical matters.

In some institutions you will have access to courses on teaching methods. Overcome your natural reticence and enrol. It is likely that one component of the course will give you the opportunity of viewing your teaching technique on video. The unit running the course may also provide an individual to come and observe your teaching, giving you the expert feedback you may not always get from a colleague.

Some personal considerations about anxiety when teaching large groups

When you are satisfied that you have attended adequately to the kinds of things discussed above, you will find it helpful to reflect on some matters of personal preparation for your teaching. Paramount among these considerations is dealing with nervousness – both before and during your large group session.

Most teachers, speakers and actors confess to feeling anxious before 'going on-stage'. However, if you are thoroughly prepared, much of the potential for nervousness will have been eliminated. And you should keep in mind that a certain level of anxiety is desirable to ensure that you perform well!

One writer on higher education, Christine Overall, has described the commonly experienced anxiety in terms of 'feeling fraudulent'. She suggests a way of managing this feeling is to act as if you know what you are doing, and to display the confidence and authority to do what you need to do. In the large group session, this may mean looking at the audience, smiling, handling audiovisual equipment confidently, being very clear and firm about instructions for active learning tasks, knowing what you will say and do at the beginning and ending of your session, and so on.

Apart from being thoroughly prepared, there are a number of 'do's and don'ts' to keep in mind.

- Do not allow yourself to conjure up visions of mistakes and disasters. Think positively. Imagine an interested and appreciative audience, achievement of the goals you set for yourself and your students, and being in control of the situation.
- Practise some relaxation exercises and deep breathing. Consult one of the numerous booklets or cassettes on this topic or attend a relaxation class if you think it might help.
- If you can, plan on arriving at the lecture room early enough to ensure everything is in order and to allow time to talk to one or two of the students in the class about their work. This approach not only serves as a valuable 'bridge' between you and your students, but also can be very helpful in meeting some of their needs and understanding difficulties that you might be able to incorporate into your teaching.

WHAT ACTIVE LEARNING STRATEGIES ARE AVAILABLE?

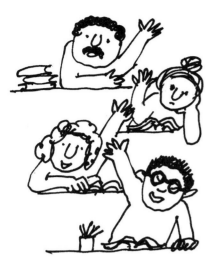

Active learning stands in contrast to much of what passes for 'learning' in large lecture classes – it is lively, dynamic, engaging and full of life. It is a basis from which lifelong learning skills can be developed. Active learning is often defined in contrast to the worst of traditional teaching where the teacher is active and the student is the passive recipient. Specifically, active learning occurs when you use strategies to ensure the session includes elements of student activity such as talking, reading, writing, thinking, or doing something. These activities might be undertaken alone, in pairs of students, or in small groups of up to about four.

There are several levels at which we would encourage you to plan for student activity. At its most basic level, we have already stressed how variety in the presentation is essential in maintaining attention and therefore the possibility of engaging with the material.

Variations in your manner and style

It is important that you feel comfortable with the way you present your session. However, you should not limit your manner and style. Changes in the volume and rate of speech, the use of silence, the maintenance of eye contact with the class and movement away from the lectern to create a less formal relationship should all be considered.

Active participation

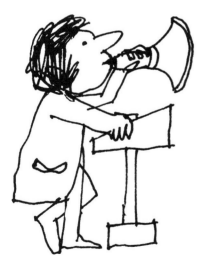

A powerful way of enhancing learning is to devise situations that require the students to interact with you or with each other. Questions are the simplest form of interaction. Many teachers ask for questions at the end of their presentation but most are disappointed in the student response. Others direct questions at students but unless the teacher is very careful, the dominant emotion will be one of fear. It is therefore preferable to create a situation in which all students answer the questions and individuals are not placed in the spotlight.

You may wish to prepare a question in the form of a multiple-choice or true-false item that can be projected as a slide or an overhead transparency. Asking for a show of hands for each alternative answer to the question can check understanding. You should follow up by explaining why each alternative is or is not a suitable answer. The time required for this will usually be about 5-7 minutes (1-2 minutes to answer the question, 4-5 minutes to give feedback on the correct and incorrect answers).

An alternative is having students ask questions. Again, if you ask 'are there any questions?' silence is the likely response because individuals do not generally like to be the focus of attention, particularly in very large classes. But if you ask students to write a question on paper and turn it in, you can then address some or all of these in a relatively anonymous and non threatening way.

Small group activity within a large group is uncommonly attempted even though it is simple to arrange for a large number of students in a theatre of any size. Once you try it out you may find it so exciting to hear the steady hum of students actually discussing your subject that you will never again feel comfortable giving a didactic lecture! The general approach is to break down the class into small groups, using a judicious rearrangement of seating if necessary. Small groups of two to four people may be formed among neighbours without any movement while larger groups may be quickly formed by two to four students in one row turning to form a group with students in the row behind. If a substantial amount of discussion time is planned the groups might best be formed at the beginning of the session and asked to spread themselves out to use up the whole lecture theatre space. The selection of the most appropriate grouping will largely depend on what you wish to achieve. Small groups may be asked to discuss a limited topic for a few minutes (sometimes called buzz groups) or to consider broader topics for a longer period of time. You may then wish to allow all or some of the groups to report back to you. This is a very useful exercise when problems are given to the students to solve and where a variety of different responses can be expected. Some more specific examples of small group activity are now discussed.

One-to-one discussion is a particularly valuable technique in the situation where you might wish all the class to consider a very emotive or challenging concept. This method is described in detail in Chapter 3 on Small Group Teaching.

Reading or problem-solving activities may be introduced. These can involve a combination of individual study and small group discussion. There are many variations on this strategy.

One example is the situation in which students are provided with an extract or article from a medical journal, a summary, a quotation, a set of diagrams or a set of clinical results. A directed-reading or problem solving task is set. This task should involve the students for 5-10 minutes. At the end of this period of individual work students are instructed to discuss something with the person beside them. They may, for instance, be asked to compare answers, draw conclusions, raise issues, identify mis-understandings or make evaluative judgements. The students are then asked for feedback. Depending on the size of the group, you could ask for reports from all or some of the pairs, have pairs report to another pair and seek general reports from these larger groups, or have a show of hands to questions or issues you have identified as you moved around the class during the discussion phase. Alternatively you could ask students to write responses, then collect these, and collate the information after the session as a basis for your teaching in the next session. Conclude by drawing ideas together, summing-up, or whatever is appropriate to the task you set them.

Whatever you do – and this is critical – thoroughly plan the activity: clearly structure the time and the tasks set, and stick to your plan (unless there are very good reasons to change). Your instructions, including the time available and tasks to be carried out, should be clearly displayed on a handout, or on the board, for ready reference during the exercise.

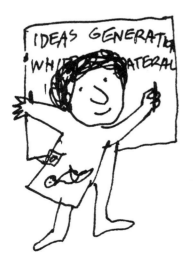

Brainstorming is a technique which can be modified for use in large group teaching. It can be of value at the beginning to stimulate interest in the topic to be discussed. The students are presented with an issue or a problem and asked to contribute as many ideas or solutions as they can. All contributions are accepted without comment or judgement as to their merits and are written on the board or on an overhead transparency. This approach encourages 'lateral' or 'divergent' thinking. One of us has successfully used this technique with a class of 120 at the beginning of a lecture. The session commenced with a request for the class to put forward their suggestions in response to a question. These suggestions were then categorised and used as a basis for further discussion in an environment where the students had been the initiators of the discussion points. Brainstorming is discussed further in the chapter on small group teaching.

Classroom Assessment Techniques (CATs) are a relatively recent innovation that we would encourage you to use with your students. These techniques stimulate active learning but most importantly help teachers gather useful information on what, how much, and how well their students are learning. The simplest and most popular CAT is the 'minute paper'. In this technique, the teacher stops two or three minutes early and asks students to write anonymous brief response to a question such as: ''What was the most important thing you learned in this class?'' or ''What important question remains unanswered?'' Papers are collected and reviewed by the teacher prior to the next class meeting at which time feedback may be given or points clarified.

Another CAT is the 'pro and con grid'. This technique assists in the development of thinking skills by encouraging students to go beyond initial reactions to an issue. In response to a suitable prompt or question, students write out a specified number of pros and cons or advantages and disadvantages. These can then be discussed in small groups, analysed in class, or analysed yourself prior to the next class session. We strongly recommend the book by Angelo and Cross on classroom assessment.

Student note-taking

The research in this area generally supports the view that note taking should be encouraged. It is a process which requires student attention and activity. The teacher can assist this process by providing a structure for material that is complex. Diagrams and other schematic representations may be more valuable than simple prose.

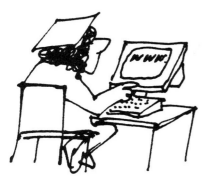

USING TEACHING MATERIALS AND TECHNOLOGY

Educational issues and the technical aspects of preparing and using teaching aids and materials are discussed in detail in Chapter 9. This section will review their use in large group teaching for a variety of purposes including illustrating the structure, providing information and examples, stimulating interest and activity, and providing variety. The aids most likely to be used are handouts, the board, overhead transparencies, slides, videos and, increasingly, on-line Internet sessions.

Handouts must serve a clear purpose and be used during the teaching session so that students are familiar with their content and simply do not file them away. Handouts may be valuable as a guide to the structure of your session and in this case may be very similar in content to the teaching plan. Such a handout should be given out at the beginning. You may wish to use the handout to provide detailed information on an area not well covered in standard student texts or not covered in detail in your teaching. Such handouts might be given out at the end of the session. Handouts may also be used to guide further study and to provide references for additional reading. Whenever you distribute handouts, it is essential that you use them in some way with your students.

'Blackboards' (which are usually green these days) and **whiteboards** are still very widely used and we urge you to look at the information in Chapter 9 about their preparation and use. Clear, legible and well-planned use of these basic aids is a delight to see and remain valuable allies in assisting you to communicate with your students. They are especially worthwhile for displaying an outline of your session or for recording feedback from students in response to questions you may have raised.

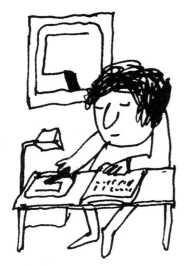

The **overhead projector** is extensively used in teaching and is particularly useful for giving outlines and listing key points. A blank sheet of paper can be used to reveal the points in sequence. A pen or pencil placed on the transparency itself should be used to direct the students' attention to the appropriate point rather than using the pointer on the screen. Information may be added with a felt pen to the transparency as the teaching proceeds. We have found that the value of the overhead is seriously reduced by four common practices. First, too much information is included on each transparency. Secondly, the teacher works through the material too quickly or talks about something different while students are trying to read and take notes from the screen. Thirdly, the transparency is carelessly positioned or is out of focus. Fourthly, and the most common abuse, is that material on transparencies is far too small to be read by students.

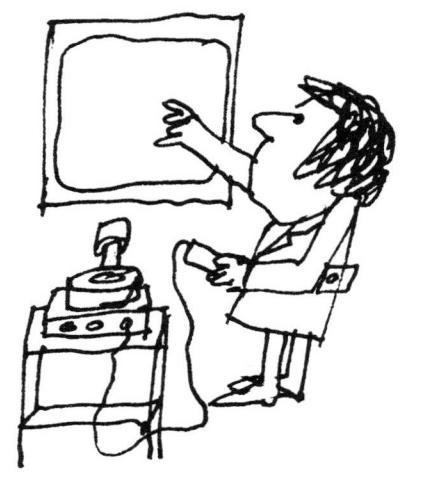

The **35-mm projector** is still widely used and some teachers build up an extensive collection of slides. However, many teachers are now incorporating their slides into Power-Point® presentations. Slides too are often misused. Those containing printed material should be kept simple and must be clearly visible at the back of the theatre with the lights on. Care must be taken when reproducing material from books and journals, which often contain far too much information. Coloured slides of relevant material are ideal for illustrating points and for adding variety and interest. When using slides, avoid turning off the lights for more than brief periods. The level of attention will rapidly fall, however interesting your slides happen to be.

Computer presentation systems (e.g. PowerPoint®) are rapidly taking over the function performed by both the overhead and slide projectors. If you teach in locations where you are confident of the technology then there are many advantages in using this aid including ease and flexibility of preparation and the capacity to generate student notes derived directly from your presentation. You can also incorporate video and sound in your presentation as required. In Chapter 9 we give you more information about preparing and using these systems.

A computer presentation is governed by the same principles as those for slides and overheads – clear, legible text and pictures, and use in a room where sufficient lighting can be left on for student note-taking and activities. If you are not confident of the environment in which you are teaching and in case the technology fails, it is still wise to have overhead transparencies or slide backups.

Videos, and less often films these days, are best utilised in short segments. Their use requires more careful planning, as it will be necessary to have a technician to set up equipment. However, the effort is well worthwhile for both the impact of the content and the variety it introduces. We use such material to show illustrative examples and practical techniques. They may also be used in attempts to influence attitudes or to explore emotionally charged issues. A short segment (trigger) can be shown illustrating some challenging situation and the class asked to react to this situation. Videos and films for this purpose are commercially available in some disciplines.

WHEN THINGS GO WRONG

Throughout this book we present the view that things are less likely to go 'wrong' if you have carefully prepared yourself for the teaching task. However, unexpected difficulties can and do arise, so strategies to deal with these need to be part of your teaching skills. In our experience problems in teaching large groups are likely to fall into one of the following categories.

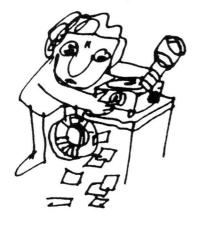

Problems with audio-visual materials and equipment. An equipment failure can be a potential disaster if you have prepared a computer presentation or a series of slides or transparencies for projection. Preventive measures include having a thorough understanding of your equipment, back-up equipment on hand, and learning to change blown bulbs or remove jammed slides.

If these measures are of no avail, you will have to continue on without the materials and may do so successfully provided that you have taken care to have a clear record in your notes of the content of your material. Photocopied enlargements of slides of data are a useful backup here. You may then be able to present some of the information verbally, on a blackboard or whiteboard, or on an overhead transparency if the original problem was with the slide projector. You will not, of course, be able to use this approach with illustrations and you may have to substitute careful description and perhaps blackboard sketches to cover essential material. Whatever you do, do not pass around your materials, which may be damaged and, of course, by the time most of the audience receive them, they are no longer directly relevant to what you are saying!

Difficulties with your presentation. Losing your place and running out of time can be disconcerting. Do not start apologising or communicate your sense of 'panic' if this should happen. Instead, pause, calmly evaluate your situation, decide on a course of action, and continue. One lecturer we know invites students to check their notes while she simply cleans the board as she thinks through what to do next!

Challenges from students. We have deliberately avoided the use of the word 'problem' in relation to your interaction with students because the 'problem' may be with you (that is, your manner, your preparation or presentation, for example) or it could be more in the form of a genuinely motivated intellectual challenge to what you have been doing or saying. It is essential to be clear as to exactly what the challenge is and why it has occurred before you act.

Many teachers fear confrontation with students in a class. We cannot go into all aspects of classroom management and discipline here, but we can identify a number of principles and refer you to more detailed discussions elsewhere (*McKeachie's Teaching Tips* is a useful reference).

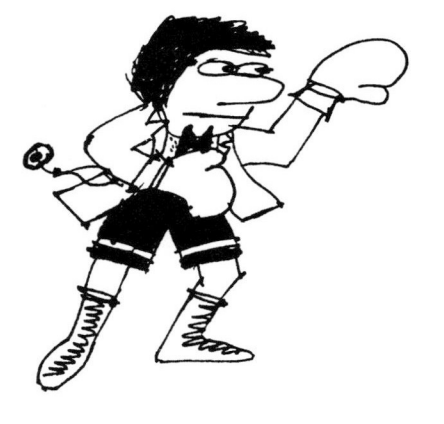

Disruptive behaviour and talking in class are common challenges and must not be ignored, both for the sake of your own concentration and for the majority of students who are there to learn. Simply stopping talking and waiting patiently for quiet usually overcomes minor disturbances. If this happens more than once the other students will usually make their displeasure known to the offenders. If the disruption is more serious, you will have to speak directly to the students concerned and indicate that you are aware of the offence. But do try initially to treat it with humour or you may alienate the rest of the class. If the problem persists, indicate that you will be unable to tolerate the situation again and that you will have to ask them to leave. Make sure you do just this if the problem re-emerges. Do so firmly and calmly. If the situation leads to confrontation, it is probably best if you leave the room. It is remarkable what effect this has on students! Make every attempt to meet the offenders afterwards to deal with the problem.

We have been appalled at accounts of teachers who endure the most unreasonable physical and verbal abuse in classes and do nothing about it – other than suffer inwardly. There is no need for this and the majority of students will look for firm but fair disciplinary measures. An added measure is to arrange arriving and leaving classes so that you have time to get to know at least some of the students in the class – especially potentially trouble-some ones. The active learning strategies we have suggested in this chapter are also ways of addressing these challenges – both by engaging students in their own learning (and using up some of their energy in this way!) and giving you a further opportunity to get to know them. Anonymity is a great accomplice in disruptive behaviour!

EVALUATING LARGE GROUP TEACHING

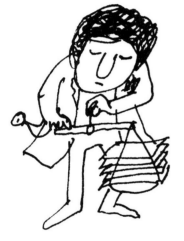

Improving the quality of your teaching in large groups will depend on a combination of experience and your willingness to critically evaluate your performance. Evaluation may be seen as informal or formal. The informal way may involve asking several students whom you know for their comments. It may also be undertaken by asking yourself a series of questions immediately after your teaching, such as:

- How much time was taken to prepare?
- Were the notes helpful?
- Were the visual aids clear and easy to read?
- What steps could be taken to improve preparation and organisation of the active learning tasks?
- Did the questions stimulate discussion?
- What did I learn about students understanding from their questions/comments/written responses to the CATs?
- Were the purposes of the session achieved? How do I know this?

The distribution of questionnaires to the class is a more formal way of evaluating teaching. Many such forms have been designed and can usually be obtained from the teaching unit within your institution. The best way of obtaining an independent evaluation is to seek the services of a teaching unit. They will sit in on your teaching and prepare a detailed analysis and go over it with you later.

A CONCLUDING THOUGHT – IF YOU MUST 'LECTURE' . . .

It may be objected that the crowded curriculum does not allow time for the active learning techniques described in this chapter. This objection rests on the view that material has to be 'covered'. However, this argument presumes that students will learn the material covered and this is unfortunately not usually the case. We have already shown that levels of attention to a traditional expository lecture decline and it is known that other indicators of performance, such as recall, fall fairly rapidly around 20 minutes after the lecture begins. Worse, what little is learned in the remainder of the lecture time interferes with understanding of material presented earlier.

So, if you feel the inclination to 'lecture' so that you have covered the material, perhaps the question you should be asking yourself is 'Should I be wasting so much time speaking for 50 minutes?' In some courses it is the case that a few students regard lectures as an important learning activity. Further, lectures are perceived as being a means to pace study, as a way of keeping in touch with the coursework, and as a supplement to other more important learning activities such as practical classes, tutorials and assignments. At worst, lectures are seen as a boring waste of time relieved only by the skill and daring of the paper plane throwers and other attention seekers!

The challenge is to work out a clear and educationally defensible rationale for lecturing. Lecturing can only be a useful *learning* method for students where the techniques of teaching large groups are appropriately employed. We hope that this chapter has contributed to dealing with these challenges.

GUIDED READING

Almost all books which are concerned with the practicalities of teaching in higher education will devote some space to the lecture method or teaching large numbers of students and you will undoubtedly find many of these helpful.

Perhaps the most popular book on lecturing is D. Bligh's *What's the Use of Lectures?*, Jossey-Bass, 2000. This book

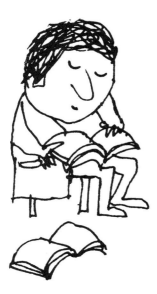

gives an overview of the research, useful information on preparing and delivering lectures, and an interesting section on alternatives to the lecture.

Another source of practical advice is the HERDSA Green Guide (No 7, 1992) *Lecturing* by R. Cannon. It includes more detail than provided in this chapter on preparation, presentation, evaluation and active learning methods. (It is available from the Higher Education Research and Development Society of Australasia, HERDSA, PO Box 516, Jamieson, ACT 2614, Australia.)

Another useful book to review for ideas on improving learning from lectures is *53 Interesting Things to Do in Your Lecture* by G. Gibbs, Technical and Educational Services Ltd, Bristol, 1992.

There is also a large published literature on active learning in large groups. A good introduction to this concept is *Promoting Active Learning* by C. Meyers and T. Jones, Jossey-Bass, San Francisco, 1993.

Books and journals referred to in this chapter:

T. Angelo and K. Cross. *Classroom Assessment Techniques: A Handbook for College Teachers*, Jossey Bass, San Francisco, 1993.

W. McKeachie. *McKeachie's Teaching Tips: Strategies, Research, and Theory for College and University Teachers*, Houghton Mifflin Co, Boston, 1998.

J. Ware and R. Williams (1975). 'The Doctor Fox Effect': A study of lecturer effectiveness and rating of instruction, *Journal of Medical Education*, **50**, 149-156.

3: TEACHING IN SMALL GROUPS

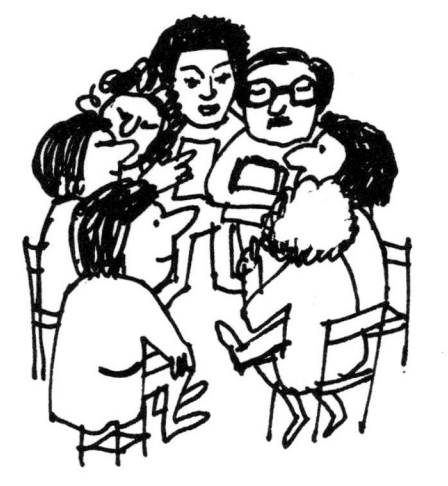

INTRODUCTION

Small group teaching can be a most rewarding experience for both teacher and student. To achieve success you will need to plan carefully and develop skills in group management. You should avoid the common error of believing that constructive discussion in groups will happen spontaneously. To avoid difficulties you will need an understanding of how groups work and how to apply a range of small group techniques to achieve the goals you set out to achieve.

THE IMPORTANCE OF SMALL GROUP TEACHING

Teaching in small groups enjoys an important place among the teaching methods commonly found in medical education for two rather different reasons. The first of these can be described as **social** and the other as **educational**. For many students in the university, and especially those in the early years of their studies, the small group or tutorial provides an important social contact with peers and teachers. The value of this contact should not be underestimated as a means for students to meet and deal with people and to resolve a range of matters indirectly associated with your teaching, such as difficulties with studying, course attendance and so on. Such matters will, of course, assist with the attainment of the educational objectives of your course.

Among the educational objectives that you can best achieve through the use of small group teaching methods are the development of higher-level intellectual skills such as reasoning and problem-solving; the development of attitudes; and the acquisition of interpersonal skills such as listening, speaking, arguing, and group leadership. Increasingly, students will need these skills so that they can participate effectively in **problem-based learning** (see Chapter 7). These skills are also important to medical students who will eventually become involved professionally with patients, other health care professionals, community groups, learned societies and the like. The distinction between social and educational aspects of small group teaching is rather an arbitrary one but it is important to bear it in mind when you plan for small group teaching.

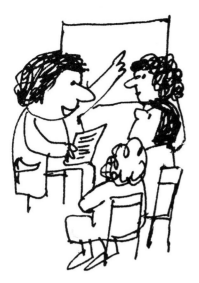

WHAT IS SMALL GROUP TEACHING?

Much of what passes for small group teaching in medical schools turns out to be little more than a lecture to a small number of students. We believe that small group teaching must have at least the following three characteristics:

➡ Active participation
➡ Face-to-face contact
➡ Purposeful activity

Active participation

The first, and perhaps the most important, characteristic of small group teaching is that teaching and learning is brought about through discussion among **all** present. This generally implies a group size that is sufficiently small to enable each group member to contribute. Research and practical experience has established that between five and eight students is ideal for most small group teaching. You will know that many so-called small groups or tutorial groups are very much larger than this ideal. Although a group of over twenty students hardly qualifies as a small group it is worth remembering that, with a little ingenuity, you can use many of the small group teaching procedures described in this chapter with considerable success with larger numbers of students. Generally speaking, though, you will be looking for a technique which allows you to break such numbers down into subgroups for at least some of the time.

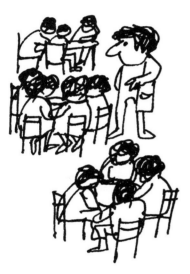

Face-to-face contact

The second characteristic of small group teaching is that it involves face-to-face contact among all those present. You will find it difficult to conduct satisfactory small group teaching in a lecture theatre or tutorial room with students sitting in rows. Similarly, long board-room type tables are quite unsuitable because those present cannot see all other group members, especially those seated alongside. Effective discussion requires communication which is not only verbal but also non-verbal involving, for example, gestures, facial expressions, eye contact and posture. This will only be achieved by sitting the group in a circle.

Purposeful activity

The third characteristic of small group teaching is that the session must have a purpose. It is certainly not an occasion for idle conversation although, regrettably, some teaching in groups appears to be little more than this. The purposes you set for your small group can be quite wide. They include discussing a topic or a patient problem and developing skills such as criticising, analysing, problem-solving and decision making. It is highly likely that you will wish the small group session to achieve more than one purpose. In medical schools, most groups are expected to deal with a substantial amount of content. However, you will also wish to use the small group approach to develop the higher intellectual skills of your students and even to influence their attitudes. In order to achieve these various purposes you will need considerable skills in managing the group and a clear plan so that discussion will proceed in an orderly fashion towards its conclusion.

MANAGING A SMALL GROUP

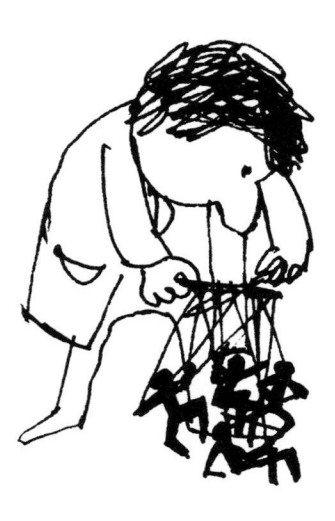

Small group teaching is considerably more challenging to manage than a conventional lecture because you must take account of the students' behaviour, personalities and the emotional aspects of being in a group. To achieve success with a small group you must also have a clear understanding of how a group operates and how it develops. You have particular responsibilities as the initial leader of the group but your role will vary considerably both within a session and from session to session. For instance, if you adopt an autocratic or authoritarian style of leadership (not an uncommon one among medical teachers) you may well have a lot of purposeful activity but there will be a limited amount of spontaneous participation. You should preferably adopt a more co-operative role where you demonstrate an expectation that the students will take responsibility for initiating discussion, providing information, asking questions, challenging statements, asking for clarification and so on. A successful group is one that can proceed purposefully without the need for constant intervention by the teacher. This is hard for most teachers to accept but is very rewarding if one recognises that this independence is one of the key goals of small group teaching and is more important than satisfying one's own need to be deferred to as teacher and content expert.

In managing a group there are two main factors that have to be considered. These are factors relating to the **task** of the group and factors relating to the **maintenance** of the group. In addition there must be a concern for the needs of each student within the group.

The tasks of the group: clear definition of tasks is something that must be high on the agenda of the first meeting. The reason for the small group sessions and their purpose in the course must be explained. In addition, you should initiate a discussion about how you wish the group to operate, what degree of preparation you expect between group meetings, what role you intend to adopt, what roles you expect the students to assume and so on. Because such details may be quickly forgotten it is desirable to provide the students with a handout. The list of headings in Figure 3.1 may be helpful:

FIGURE 3.1.
SUGGESTED HEADINGS FOR A
SMALL GROUP HANDOUT

- Course title, description and aims.
- Teacher's name and availability.
- List of students' names.
- How the group is to run (e.g. teacher's role, students' roles, method to be used).
- Work requirements (e.g. assignments, case presentations).
- Assessment arrangements.
- Reading matter.

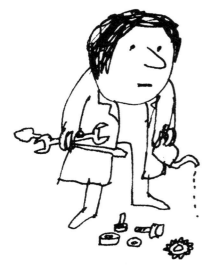

Maintenance of the group: this refers to the achievement of a good 'climate' for discussion. Ideally it is one that is open, trustful and supportive rather than closed, suspicious, defensive and competitive. It is important to establish that the responsibility for group maintenance rests with the students as well as with the teacher. The firm but pleasant handling of the loquacious or dominating students early in the session or the encouragement of the quiet student are obvious examples of what can be achieved to produce the required environment for effective group discussion.

The successfully managed group will meet the criteria shown in Figure 3.2.

FIGURE 3.2.
CRITERIA FOR A GOOD GROUP
(AFTER HILL, 1982)

- Prevalence of a warm, accepting, non-threatening group climate.
- Learning approached as a co-operative rather than a competitive enterprise.
- Learning accepted as the major reason for the existence of the group.
- Active participation by all.
- Equal distribution of leadership functions.
- Group sessions and learning tasks are enjoyable.
- Content adequately and efficiently covered.
- Evaluation accepted as an integral part of the group's activities.
- Students attend regularly.
- Students come prepared.

STRUCTURE IN SMALL GROUP TEACHING

We mentioned earlier the need to have a clear plan so that the group discussion will proceed with purpose and in an orderly fashion. A structured approach to tasks and to the allocation of the time available is a useful tool for you to consider. An example of such a structured discussion session is illustrated in Figure 3.3.

FIGURE 3.3.
STRUCTURED CASE DISCUSSION
SESSION

#		
1	PRELIMINARIES/HOUSEKEEPING MATTERS	5 MINS
2	A STUDENT PRESENTS THE INITIAL HISTORY AND EXAMINATION FINDING OF A WARD PATIENT	5 MINS
3	GROUP ASKED TO GENERATE HYPOTHESES AND DIAGNOSES, DISCUSS IMMEDIATE MANAGEMENT AND INITIAL INVESTIGATIONS	15 MINS
4	INFORMATION PROVIDED ON WHAT THE STUDENT (AND CONSULTANT) THOUGHT WAS THE DIAGNOSIS, WHAT WAS DONE, AND WHICH INVESTIGATIONS WERE ORDERED. GROUP DISCUSSES ANY DISPARITIES	10 MINS
5	STUDENT PRESENTS FURTHER DATA ON INVESTIGATIONS AND PROGRESS. GROUP DISCUSSES ANY DISPARITIES	10 MINS
6	GROUP LEADER OFFERS CONCLUDING REMARKS AND OPPORTUNITY FOR CLARIFICATION OF UNRESOLVED ISSUES	5 MINS
	TOTAL	50 MINS

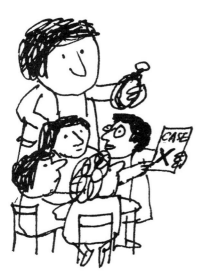

This is a structure of a discussion based on a case presentation. Note that the structure lays out what is to be discussed and how much time is budgeted. Such a scheme is not intended to encourage undue rigidity or inflexibility, but to clarify purposes and tasks. This may seem to be a trivial matter, but it is one which creates considerable uncertainty for students. Keeping to a time budget is very difficult. You need to be alert to how time is being spent and whether time for one part of the plan can be transferred to an unexpected and important issue that arises during discussion.

Another structure, not commonly used in medical education, is illustrated in Figure 3.4.

FIGURE 3.4.
A SNOWBALLING GROUP
DISCUSSION (AFTER NORTHEDGE,
1975)

INDIVIDUAL WORK	
STUDENTS READ BRIEF BACKGROUND DOCUMENT ON TOPIC, READ CASE HISTORY AND EXAMINE LABORATORY RESULTS	10 MIN
WORK IN PAIRS	
STUDENTS COMPARE UNDERSTANDINGS, CLEAR UP DIFFICULTIES, MAKE PRELIMINARY DIAGNOSIS AND DECIDE ON FURTHER TESTS	10 MIN
WORK IN SMALL GROUPS	
PAIRS REPORT TO THE SMALL GROUP. GROUP DISCUSSES DIAGNOSES AND FURTHER TESTS, SEEKING AGREEMENT OR CLARIFYING DISAGREEMENTS. GROUP PREPARES REPORT FOR WHOLE GROUP	15 MIN
REPORTING BACK TO WHOLE GROUP	
EACH SMALL GROUP PRESENTS REPORT. TEACHER NOTES MAIN POINTS ON BOARD, FLIPCHART PAPER OR OVERHEAD TRANSPARENCY. AS GROUPS CONTRIBUTE, TEACHER AND STUDENTS OFFER COMMENTS. TEACHER OR STUDENTS ATTEMPT SUMMARY OF POINTS RAISED AND SOME FORM OF CONCLUSION	20 MIN

This structure includes the principle of 'snow-balling' groups. From an individual task, the student progresses through a series of small groups of steadily increasing size. There are special advantages in using this structure which are worth noting: it does not depend on prior student preparation for its success; the initial individual work brings all students to approximately the same level before

discussion begins; and it ensures that everyone partici-
pates, at least in the preliminary stages.

INTRODUCING STIMULUS MATERIALS

A very useful means of getting discussion going in groups
is to use what is generally known as 'stimulus material'. We
have seen how this was done in the snowballing group
structure described previously. The range of stimulus
material is really very large indeed. It is limited only by
your imagination and the objectives of your course. Here
are a few examples:

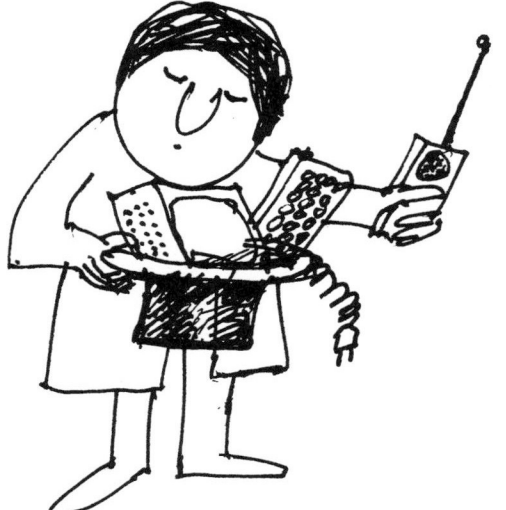

- A short multiple-choice test (ambiguous items work
  well in small groups).
- A case history.
- Video (e.g. short open-ended situation, such as a
  patient's reaction to a doctor).
- A real or simulated patient.
- Observation of a role-play.
- Visual materials (e.g. X-rays, photographs, slides,
  specimens, real objects, charts, diagrams, statistical
  data).
- An audio recording (e.g. an interview, heart sounds, a
  segment of a radio broadcast).
- A student's written report on a project or a patient.
- Computer or Web-based material.
- A journal article or other written material (an
  interesting example is provided by Moore where he
  used extracts from literary works to help students
  understand the broader cultural, philosophical, ethical
  and personal issues of being a doctor. Examples of
  sources of these extracts included Solzhenitsyn's
  Cancer Ward and Virginia Woolf's *On Being Ill*).

ALTERNATIVE SMALL GROUP DISCUSSION TECHNIQUES

As with any other aspect of teaching it is helpful to
understand several techniques in order to introduce
variety or to suit a particular situation. Such techniques
include:

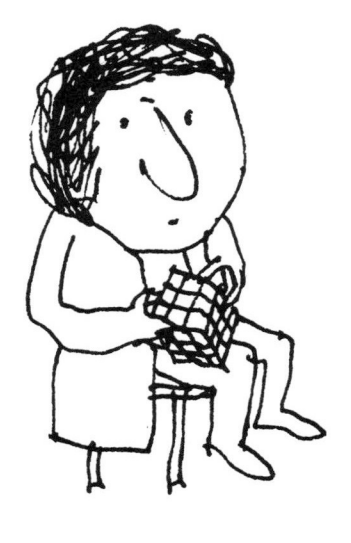

- ★ One-to-one discussion
- ★ Buzz groups
- ★ Brainstorming
- ★ Role playing
- ★ Evaluation discussion

1. One-to one discussion

This is a very effective technique which can be used with a group of almost any size. It is particularly useful as an 'ice-breaker' when the group first meets, and is valuable for enhancing listening skills. It can also be used to discuss controversial or ethical issues when forceful individuals with strong opinions need to be prevented from dominating the discussion (Figure 3.5).

FIGURE 3.5.
CONDUCTING A ONE-TO-ONE
DISCUSSION

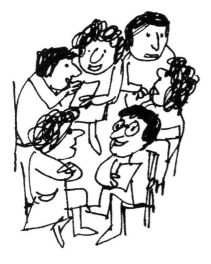

A Procedure

- Group members (including the teacher) divide into pairs and each person is designated 'A' or 'B'.
- Person A talks to person B for an uninterrupted period of 3-5 minutes on the topic for discussion.
- Person B listens and avoids prompting or questioning.
- Roles are reversed with B talking to A.
- At the conclusion the group reassembles.
- Each person, in turn, introduces themselves before introducing the person to whom they were speaking. They then briefly paraphrase what was said by that person.

B Use as icebreaker

- Group members are asked to respond to a question such as 'tell me something about yourself'.

C General use

- Group members respond to appropriate questioning, e.g. 'what is your opinion about . . . ?'

It can be useful to insist on the no interruption rule (though not so much when used as an icebreaker). Prolonged periods of silence may ensue but person A will be using this time for uninterrupted thinking, a luxury not available in most situations. Often the first superficial response to a question will be changed after deeper consideration.

Buzz groups

These are particularly helpful to encourage maximum participation at one time. It is therefore especially useful when groups are large, if too many people are trying to contribute at once or, alternatively, if shyness is inhibiting several students (Figure 3.6).

FIGURE 3.6.
CONDUCTING A BUZZ GROUP

Procedure

➡ The group is divided into subgroups of 3-4 students.
➡ Discussion occurs for a few minutes (the term 'buzz' comes from the noise of verbal activity!).
➡ A clear task must be set.
➡ Each group reports back to the whole group.

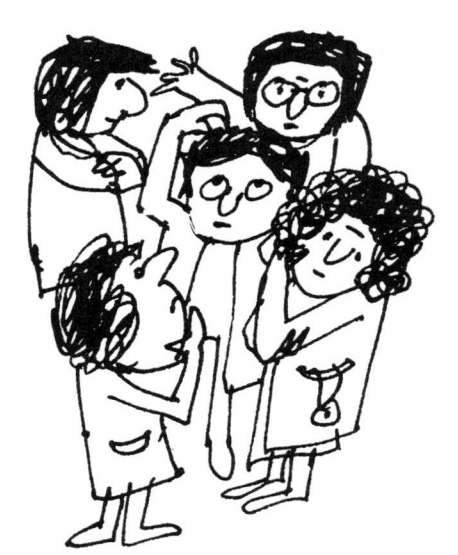

FIGURE 3.7.
CONDUCTING A BRAINSTORMING
SESSION

3. Brainstorming

This is a technique that you should consider when you wish to encourage broad and creative thinking about a problem. It is also valuable when highly critical group members (including perhaps yourself?) appear to be inhibiting discussion. If used frequently, it trains students to think up ideas before they are dismissed or criticised. The key to successful brainstorming is to separate the generation of ideas, or possible solutions to a problem, from the evaluation of these ideas or solutions (Figure 3.7)

Procedure

★ Explain the rules of brainstorming to the group:
  ● Criticism is ruled out during the idea generation stage.
  ● All ideas are welcome.
  ● Quantity of ideas is the aim (so as to improve the chances of good ideas coming up).
  ● Combination and improvement of ideas is sought.
★ State the problem to the group.
★ A period of silent thought is allowed during which students write down their ideas.
★ Ideas are then recorded (in a round robin format) on a blackboard, overhead transparency or flip-chart paper for all to see.
★ When all ideas are listed, and combination and improvement of ideas has been completed, discussion and evaluation commences.

4. Role playing

This is a powerful and underused technique. It is valuable in teaching interpersonal and communication skills, particularly in areas with a high emotional content. It has been found to be helpful in changing perceptions and in developing empathy. It is not a technique to use without some experience so you should arrange to sit in on a role play session before using it in your own course. In this regard, your colleagues teaching psychiatry or counselling should be able to help as will the Green Guide by Ernington (Figure 3.8).

FIGURE 3.8.
CONDUCTING A ROLE PLAY

Procedure

➡ Explain the nature and purpose of the exercise.
➡ Define the setting and situation.
➡ Select students to act out roles.
➡ Provide players with a realistic description of the role or even a script. Allow time for them to prepare and, if necessary, practice.
➡ Specify observational tasks for non-players.
➡ Allow sufficient time for the role play.
➡ Discuss and explore the experience with players and observers.

5. Plenary sessions

In many group teaching situations, and sometimes conferences, subgroups must report back to the larger group. This reporting back can be tedious and often involves only the subgroup leaders who may present a very distorted view of what happened. The plenary session method may help you solve these problems (Figure 3.9).

FIGURE 3.9.
CONDUCTING A PLENARY SESION

Procedure

● Subgroups sit together facing other subgroups.
● The convenor of subgroup A briefly reports the substance of the discussion of this group.
● The convenor of subgroup B then invites members of subgroups B, C, D, etc. to ask questions of any member of group A.
● After 10 minutes convenor of sub group B reports on the discussion in subgroup B
● The process is repeated for each subgroup.
● The 10 minute (or other) time limits must be adhered to strictly.

USING TECHNOLOGY FOR TEACHING SMALL GROUPS

By combining computers and communication technology, you can make fundamental changes to the way you present and distribute material and interact with your students. By using these technologies, the distinctions between large and small group teaching tend to break down.

However, some examples of the ways in which technology can be used specifically to support small group teaching are:

- By using electronic mail (e-mail) to communicate with one or more students
- Through electronic discussion groups
- By conferencing techniques using computer, sound and video.

Implementing electronic teaching is different to other approaches in many ways. For instance, uninitiated colleagues will be totally uncomprehending if you object to being interrupted when you are working at your computer by saying you are 'teaching'!

One fundamental difference between face-to-face teaching and being 'on-line' is that you will be interacting with what is known as a 'virtual' group. This means that the group does not exist as an entity at any one time or place, but that it is dispersed both in time (within limits) and place and that the group interacts 'asynchronously' at different times. Furthermore, there are different rules of behaviour for electronic communication known colloquially as 'netiquette' and which both you and your students should observe. To learn more about this topic you can search for it on the World Wide Web. A very good overview is provided at:
< http//www.albion.com/netiquette/book/index.html >
or in the book *Netiquette* by Virginia Shea.

EVALUATING SMALL GROUP TEACHING

Evaluation implies collecting information about your teaching and then making judgements based on that information. Making judgements based on what one student says, or on rumour or intuition, is simply not good enough. You must collect information in a way that is likely to lead to valid conclusions. However, constant evaluation

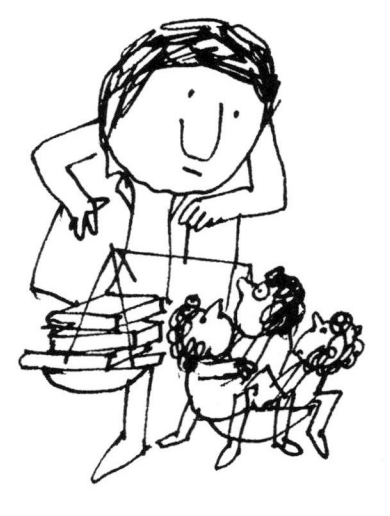

of small group activities is not recommended as it may inhibit the development and working of the group. Evaluation may be of two types: informal or formal.

Informal evaluation: this can proceed from a careful reflection on what happened during your time with the group. You may do this by considering a number of criteria which you feel are important. For example, you may be interested in the distribution of discussion among group members, the quality of contribution, the amount of time you talked, whether the purpose of the session was achieved, what students have learned, and so on. Of course, your reflections will be biased and it is wise to seek confirmation by questioning students from time to time. However, the importance of informal evaluations lies in your commitment to turn these reflections into improvements. If you are concerned with your own performance, the assistance of a trusted and experienced colleague sitting in on the group, or even just a discussion of your own feelings about the group, may be very helpful.

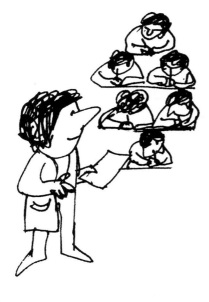

Formal evaluation: formal approaches to evaluation include the use of questionnaires or the analysis of video recordings of the group at work. Standard questionnaires are available which seek student responses to a set number of questions. An example is shown at the end of the chapter (Figure 3.10).

Although such standard questionnaires can be useful you may find it more beneficial to design one that contributes more directly to answering questions which relate to your own course and concerns. As questionnaire design can be difficult, it is recommended that you seek the assistance of a teaching unit. The analysis of videos of your group at work is also a task which would require the expertise of someone from a teaching unit.

WHEN THINGS GO WRONG

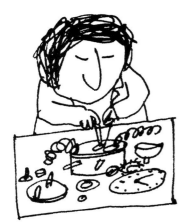

You may encounter a variety of difficulties in your group sessions. For example, while you might decide to ignore a sleeping student or an amorous couple in a lecture class, providing it was not disruptive, it would be impossible to do so in a small group. How you resolve these difficulties with the group is critical. An authoritarian approach would almost certainly destroy any chance of establishing the co-operative climate we believe to be essential. It is generally more appropriate to raise the problem with the group and ask them for their help with a solution.

One of your main roles as a group leader is to be sensitive to the group and the individuals within it. Research has identified a number of difficulties that students commonly experience. These are:

★ Making a contribution to the discussion.
★ Understanding the conventions of group work and acceptable models of behaviour.
★ Knowing enough to contribute to the discussion.
★ Being assessed.

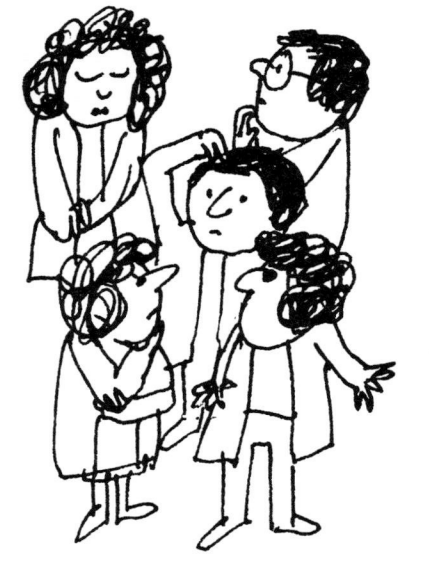

These difficulties frequently get in the way of productive discussion. They tend to be due to genuine confusion on the part of students combined with a fear of exposing their ignorance in front of the teacher and their peers. It is therefore essential for you to clarify the purpose of the group and the way in which students are to enter into the discussion. Their previous experience of small group sessions or ward teaching might lead them to see the occasion as only a threatening question and answer session. They must learn that ignorance is a relative term and that their degree of ignorance must be recognised and explored before effective learning can begin. A will-ingness by the teacher to admit ignorance and demon-strate an appropriate way of dealing with it will be very reassuring to many students.

Confusion in the students' minds about how they are being assessed can also cause difficulties. Generally speaking, assessing contributions to discussion is inhibiting and should be avoided. If you do not have discretion in this matter then at least make it quite clear what criteria you are looking for in your assessment. Should you be able to determine your own assessment policy then the following are worth considering:

➡ Require attendance at all (or a specified proportion of) group meetings as a prerequisite.
➡ Set formal written work, e.g. an essay, a series of short papers, a case analysis.
➡ Set a group-based task, e.g. keeping an account of the work done by the group.

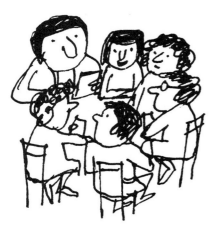

The teacher's perceptions of group difficulties may not necessarily match those of the students. A discussion with the group about how they think things are going or the administration of a short questionnaire are ways of seeking feedback.

Once the group is operating it is important to monitor progress. Be sensitive to the emotional responses of the group and to the behaviour of individual students. The book by Tiberius is a useful source of additional advice on such issues.

GUIDED READING

For a wide-ranging discussion of the purposes and techniques of small group teaching we suggest you turn to the collection of papers edited by D. Bligh: *Teach Thinking by Discussion*, SRHE/NFER, Nelson, Guildford, UK 1986. This monograph also provides a good introduction to the research literature on small groups. Also *Small Group Teaching: A Troubleshooting Guide* by R. Tiberius, Kogan Page, London, 1999.

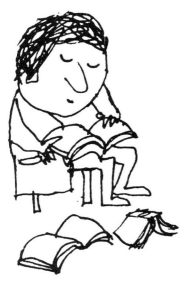

Another excellent guide, to both the theory and the practice of group work, is D. Jacques, *Learning in Groups*, Kogan Page, London 1991.

Books and journals referred to in this chapter

W. Hill. *Learning Thru Discussion*. Sage, California, 1982.

W. Bion. *Experiences in Groups*. Tavistock, London, 1968.

A. Moore (1976). Medical Humanities – A New Medical Adventure. *New England Journal of Medicine*, **295**, 1479-80.

A. Northedge (1975). Learning Through Discussion at the Open University. *Teaching at a Distance*, **2**, 10-17.

E. Ernington (1997). *Role Play*. HERDSA Green Guide No 21. (available from HERDSA, PO Box 516, Jamieson, ACT 2614, Australia).

FIGURE 3.10.
EXAMPLE OF TUTORIAL QUESTIONNAIRE (ADVISORY CENTRE FOR UNIVERSITY EDUCATION, UNIVERSITY OF ADELAIDE)

		Very Heavy			Reasonable		Very Light		N/A
1	The workload for the tutorials was …	7	6	5	4	3	2	1	X
		Strongly Agree			Undecided		Strongly Disagree		N/A
2	The tutorials were relevant to the aims of the subject	7	6	5	4	3	2	1	X
3	The tutorials were well organised	7	6	5	4	3	2	1	X
4	The number of students in the classroom was appropriate for effective participation	7	6	5	4	3	2	1	X
5	The lecture, tutorials and clinical sessions were appropriately linked	7	6	5	4	3	2	1	X
6	The tutorials were valuable for my understanding of the subject	7	6	5	4	3	2	1	X
7	The tutorials stimulated my interest in the subject	7	6	5	4	3	2	1	X
8	The tutorial work could be completed within the allocated time.	7	6	5	4	3	2	1	X
9	More guidance should have been provided on how to work in a group	7	6	5	4	3	2	1	X
10	The assessment of tutorial work was fair	7	6	5	4	3	2	1	X
11	Teacher expectations were made clear	7	6	5	4	3	2	1	X
12	I received adequate feedback on my work	7	6	5	4	3	2	1	X
13	I was able to discuss my progress	7	6	5	4	3	2	1	X
14	The recommended textbook was valuable for my understanding of the subject.	7	6	5	4	3	2	1	X
15	Resource materials were readily available	7	6	5	4	3	2	1	X
16	My involvement in the tutorials was high	7	6	5	4	3	2	1	X
17	I have developed more confidence in myself	7	6	5	4	3	2	1	X
18	I have developed skills needed by professionals in this field	7	6	5	4	3	2	1	X
19	What changes should be made to the tutorials and why?								
20	What changes should be made to the assessment procedures, and why?								

If you would like to make further comments on this subject, do so below.
Thank you for answering this questionnaire

4:   MAKING A PRESENTATION AT A CONFERENCE

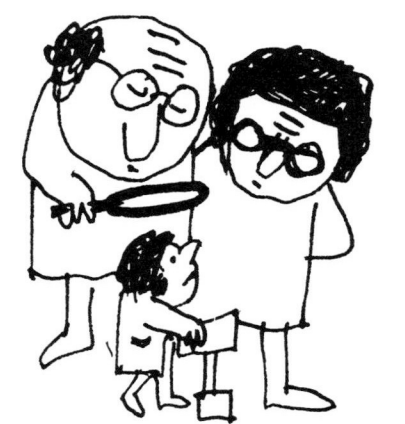

INTRODUCTION

This chapter may appear to be out of place in a book about education and teaching. However, most medical teachers, at some time, will wish to make a presentation at a scientific meeting. There are many obvious similarities between giving a lecture and presenting a paper. There are also significant differences which may not be quite so obvious which made us feel that this chapter might be appreciated.

Poster sessions are growing in popularity at many national and international meetings as an alternative to the formal presentation of papers. We have, therefore, included a short segment on the preparation of a conference poster.

PRESENTING A PAPER

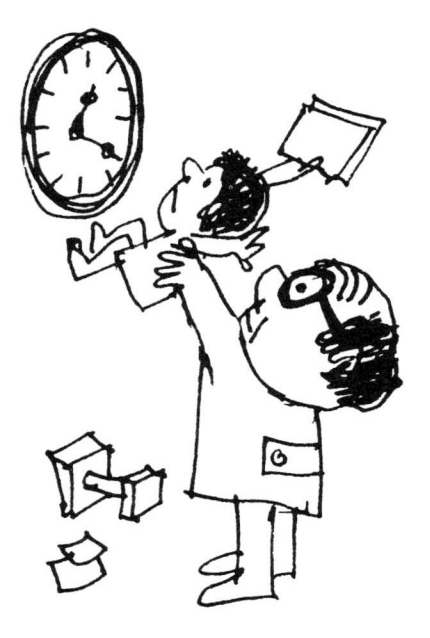

Though much of the advice given in the chapter on lecturing is just as relevant in this section, the aims of a scientific meeting or conference are different enough to warrant separate consideration. Much of this difference relates to the restriction on time. It is likely that a strict time limit will be imposed. If you are in the position to give a paper it is certain that you will have a lot to say, far more in fact than can possibly be delivered in such a short time. You will also be caught in the difficult situation of having many of the audience unfamiliar with the details of your area of interest, some of the audience knowing considerably more than you do about the area, and all of the audience likely to be critical of the content and presentation. These and other factors make the giving of a scientific paper an anxiety provoking situation, particularly for the young and inexperienced lecturer hoping to make a good impression on peers and superiors. However, it is also a situation that is amenable to resolution by careful planning and attention to technique.

PREPARING THE PAPER

Much of the advice that follows was admirably dealt with many years ago in the classic book by Calnan and Barabas entitled *Speaking at Medical Meetings*. They described three stages that you must go through during the preparation of a short scientific communication.

★ The collection and selection of the data.
★ The arrangement (getting the structure right and deciding on the most suitable visual aids).
★ Polishing, writing it out and rehearsal.

These same basic headings have been retained in this chapter.

The collection and selection of the data

There is a great tendency for speakers to cram more than is possible into their papers with the inevitable consequence of either speaking too fast or going over time. The audience knows that it is not possible to cover everything in detail and is primarily interested in hearing a short cohesive account of your research. To achieve this you are not going to be able to present all your hard-won data. You are going to have to be very selective and in most instances you will have to restrict yourself to one aspect of your work.

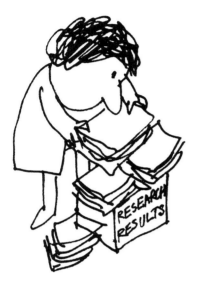

Your first step should be to write down in one sentence the main purpose of your paper. In other words, what is the main message you wish to get across? Having done this you should identify the three or four pieces of evidence you will use to give support to your views. You should keep in mind that you will only have two or three minutes to describe each piece of work so that when you are assembling your data you must be aware of the need to simplify the results into a more easily digested form (e.g. complex tables reconstructed into histograms).

The arrangement

The first task is to get the basic plan worked out. The presentation will fall into several components.

● Introduction
● Statement of the purpose of your research
● Description of methods and results
● Conclusions

The introduction: this is a vital component of your talk. It must set the context of your work for the audience, many of whom may not be experts in your field. They may also be suffering the after effects of the previous paper or of a dash from another concurrent session venue. You have no more than two minutes to excite the interest of the audience before they relapse into the mental torpor so prevalent at scientific meetings. You must therefore give a considerable amount of thought to the introduction. It must be simple, precise and free from jargon. It must start from a broad base so that the audience can identify the point at which your research fits into the scheme of things and make them appreciate the vital importance of your own contribution.

The statement of purpose: this should take no more than a minute but it is also a vital component of the talk. In these few sentences you will have to convince the audience that what you set out to do was worthwhile. It should flow from the introduction so that it sounds like a logical outcome of previous research.

The description of methods and results: the description of methods will usually have to be abbreviated or even reduced to a mention ('The so-and-so technique was used to . . .'). If the development of a new method is an important part of your work then obviously it must be described in more detail but you must decide whether the main message is to relate to the method or the results subsequently obtained.

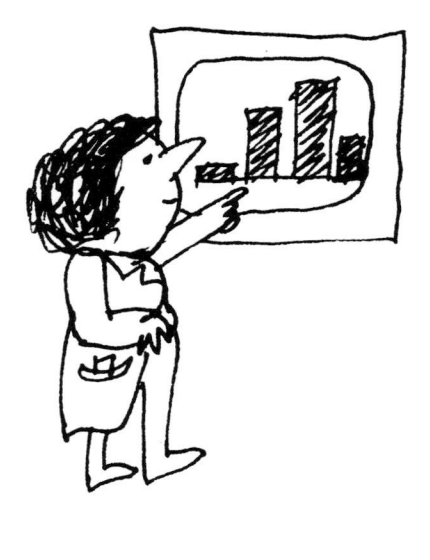

The results are usually the most important part of the paper. You will inevitably have spent a lot of time getting them together. It is possible that you have already prepared a variety of tables, graphs and charts for the purpose of publication. Do not fall into the trap of thinking that these are suitable for presentation to a live audience. How often have you, for example, sat in a meeting where someone has projected slides of an incomprehensible and illegible table taken straight from a journal!

The conclusions: these must flow naturally from the results. You will be aiming to make one or two clear statements which you are able to conclude from your work. It is advisable to be reasonably modest in your claims.

The presentation aids

The second task is to prepare the visual aids. In most instances these will be slides, overhead transparencies or a computer-based presentation. Considerable thought must be given to these as their impact and quality may make or break the presentation. They must complement your oral presentation, not duplicate it. The technical aspects of the preparation of visual materials are covered in greater detail in Chapter 9 but a few specific points are worth mentioning at this time.

Having roughed out the plan of the talk it should be reasonably obvious where a slide or overhead transparency is required. You may need one or two during the introduction, such as a clinical picture of a patient or an illustration of a previous piece of research. You may not have time to say much about the method but an illustration of the technique may be pertinent. If so, simple line diagrams are usually more valuable than photographs.

The display of the results provide you with the greatest challenge. It is during this part of your paper that the visual material will often be of more importance than the verbal explanation ('A picture says a thousand words'). Avoid complex tables and where possible convert tables to charts or simple graphs. Rarely is it appropriate to show masses of individual data, just show the mean or rounded off figures. If you feel you really must refer to complex data it is better to have this prepared in printed form and distributed to the audience.

Having prepared the illustrations, check that they are accurate and legible. As a rough rule, a slide where the information can be read with the naked eye will be satisfactory when projected. Lettering on an overhead transparency must be no less than 5 mm high and for a computer-based presentation a minimum of 32 points is suggested. Then take them to a large lecture theatre and project them. Check that they are indeed legible from the furthermost corners of the theatre. It is also helpful to take a colleague with you to check that the message is clear and that there are no spelling mistakes.

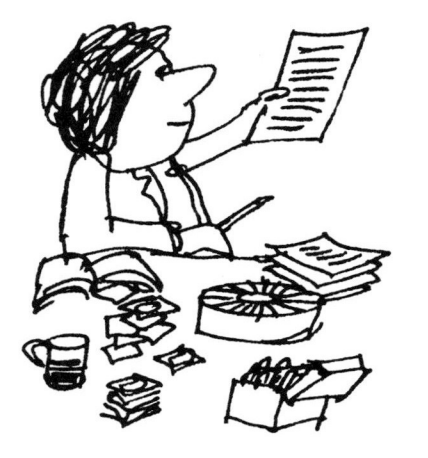

Polishing, writing it out and rehearsal

At this stage you should have a good idea of what you intend to say and the visual aids that you require. It is now advisable to write the text of the talk in full. Do not write in the style you use for journal publications. Pretend you are talking to an individual and write in a conversational mode, avoiding jargon wherever possible.

As you go along identify the correct position for the visual aids. You may find places where you have not prepared an appropriate illustration. This should be rectified even if it is only to consist of a couple of key words. Remember, during the talk the visual aids must complement your talk and not distract from it. There must always be an accurate match between the content of your aid and what you are saying. If you do not have an aid to illustrate what you are saying, insert a blank rather than leaving on an irrelevant illustration.

Once you have the rough draft, edit it. Then read it aloud at about the pace you think you will go during the presentation. Further editing and alterations will be required, as almost certainly you will have gone over time. Some find it a useful ploy at this stage to record the talk on a tape recorder and listen to the result very critically.

The next stage is to present the paper to an honest and critical colleague. The feedback is often extremely valuable. At this state you will have finalised the text and aids.

You must now make the decision whether you will read the paper or not. Most authorities consider that you should be well enough rehearsed to speak only with the aid of cue cards or the cues provided by your visual aids. If you have a highly visual presentation most of the audience will be looking at the screen so the fact that you are reading is less critical. Providing the text is written in conversational style, and you are able to look up from the text at frequent intervals, then reading is not a major sin. The chief risk of speaking without a text in a very short presentation is going over time which at best will irritate the chair and the audience, and at worst will result in your being cut off in mid-sentence.

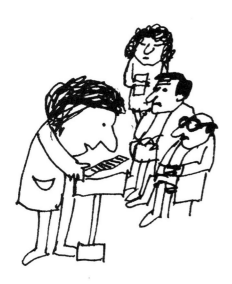

Whatever you decide, rehearsal is essential and a dress rehearsal in front of an audience (e.g. the department) a week or two before the event is invaluable. Not only will you receive comments on the presentation but you will also be subject to questions, the answering of which, in a precise manner, is just as important as the talk itself.

PREPARING THE ABSTRACT AND YOUR CONTRIBUTION TO THE PROCEEDINGS OF THE CONFERENCE

The abstract

Most conferences will require you to prepare an abstract, sometimes several months before the meeting. It may initially be used to help select contributions and will ultimately be made available to participants. Contributors are often tardy in preparing their abstracts which is discourteous to the conference organisers and makes their task more difficult.

The abstract should be an advertisement for your paper. It should outline the background to the study and summarise the supporting data and the main conclusions. Quite frequently abstracts promise what they do not deliver so avoid becoming guilty of false advertising.

The proceedings

Many national and most major international conferences will publish proceedings. Should you be presenting a paper as such a conference you will be required to provide your contribution to these proceedings during the conference or shortly afterwards. It is not appropriate to present the organisers with the script and slides that you have just used in your presentation. The contribution to the proceedings should be written in a style consistent with that used in a journal article. The content should be the same as in the presented paper but not necessarily identical. It is perfectly permissible to expand some areas, particularly with regard to the methods and results sections, where more details could be included. This should, of course, all be done within the guidelines for format and length specified by the organisers.

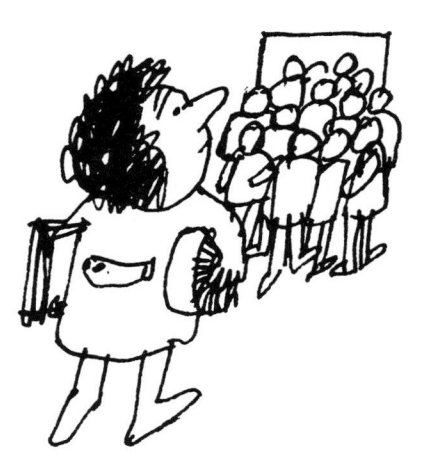

WHAT YOU SHOULD DO ON THE DAY

'There's many a slip twixt cup and lip'. This saying provides a reminder that, however good your preparation for the presentation of the paper has been, there is still plenty that can happen to ruin your carefully laid plans. Fortunately, many such problems can be prevented or anticipated. You should find it useful to work your way through the checklist in Figure 4.1.

Handling questions

Most conferences have a fixed period of time for questions. In some ways this is the most critical part of the presentation. Some people in the audience are going to test you out with penetrating questions and how you handle them will enhance or detract from the impact of your performance. This is one of the reasons why we suggested a full dress rehearsal in front of your department in order to practice your answering of difficult questions for which some participants will be eagerly searching. The following are some points to remember:

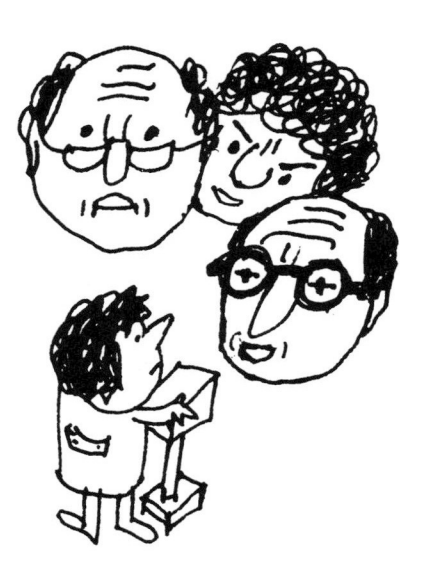

★ Listen to the question very carefully.
★ If the question is complex or if you suspect that not all the audience heard it, restate it clearly and succinctly.
★ Answer the question politely and precisely. Sometimes a simple 'yes' or 'no' will be sufficient. Avoid the danger of using the question to give what amounts to a second paper.
★ Be alert to questioners who are deliberately trying to trick you or to use the occasion to display their own knowledge of the subject.
★ If the question is particularly awkward or aggressive try to deflect it as best you can. Strategies include agreeing with as much of what was said as possible, acknowledging legitimate differences of opinion or interpretation, or suggesting you meet the questioner afterwards to clarify your position. At all costs avoid a heated head-on clash in front of your audience. However, do not be afraid to politely disagree with any questioners, however eminent, when you are sure of your ground. Remember, they may only be testing you out.

FIGURE 4.1.
CHECKLIST TO USE ON THE DAY OF
THE PRESENTATION

Before the presentation

★ Check your slides or overheads to see that they are in the correct order, labelled in this order and if slides are used, spotted in the correct place (see Figure 9.4).

★ Load your slides or boot up your computer slide show. Project them to double check that they are in the correct order and be sure you can operate the equipment with confidence.

★ Seek out the technician and explain your plan for the slides and the arrangements for lighting.

★ Check your prompt cards or text.

★ Check the venue and audio-visual facilities. You may be expected to operate the lights, a computer, a slide changer and a light pointer. Have a practice during a break in the programme.

★ If you are expected to use a microphone check how it is attached or adjusted.

★ Try and sit in on a talk in the same venue early in the day to get a feel for the acoustics and how you should use the audio-visual facilities.

During the presentation

★ Walk confidently to the podium and arrange your cards or text. Adjust the microphone and set out the position of pointers, transparencies, slide changers and so on to your satisfaction.

★ Commence your talk with an appropriate opening.

★ Present the opening few sentences without reference to any notes, looking around the audience without fixing your eyes on any particular individual, however friendly or prestigious that person may be.

★ Call for the lights to be dimmed (or do it yourself) when your first slide is to appear. Never turn off the lights completely unless it is absolutely essential and in any case only for a minimum of time. On the other hand do not continually call for 'lights on' or 'lights off'. Your slides should have been designed to be clearly visible in subdued light.

★ Speak at a rate which sounds slow to you – it will not be too slow for the audience. Try and use more emphasis than seems natural to your own ear – again, it will not sound too theatrical to the audience. Let your enthusiasm show through by using suitable hand and facial gestures.

★ When you turn to the screen to point something out make sure you do not move away from the microphone. This is a particular problem with a fixed microphone, in which case move behind it so your continue to speak across it.

● When you come to the conclusion, say so ('In conclusion, I have shown . . . or finally . . .').

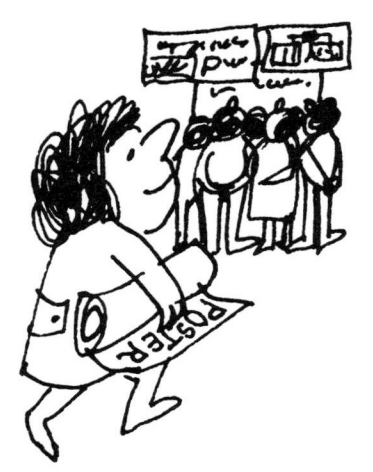

PREPARING A CONFERENCE POSTER

The conference poster is an increasingly popular alternative to presenting papers at conferences. You will find that the poster has several advantages over the traditional paper such as:

➡ Allowing readers to consider material at their own rate.
➡ Being available for viewing over an extended period of time.
➡ Enabling participants to engage in more detailed discussion with the presenter than is the case with the usually rushed paper discussion session.

If the conference organisers have arranged a poster session we suggest that you consider taking advantage of it. It may provide you with an opportunity to present additional material to the conference that would otherwise be difficult because of limitations on the number of speakers.

What is a conference poster?

A conference poster is a means of presenting information from a static display. A poster should include a least the following parts:

★ A title
★ An abstract
★ Text and diagrams
★ Name of author(s), their address(es) and where they may be contacted during the conference.

Additional material that you might consider for the poster, or in support of the poster, includes:

● Illustrations and photographs
● Exhibits and objects
● Audio-visual displays, such as a video
● A take-away handout, which might be a printed reduction of your poster.
● A blank pad, so that when you are not in attendance interested readers can leave comments or contact addresses for follow-up.

Preparing the poster

If you decide that a poster is an appropriate way of presenting your information, there are a number of things you must take into consideration during its presentation.

Firstly, ascertain from the conference organisers the facilities and size of space that will be available. Then proceed to plan the poster. The poster should communicate your message as simply as possible, so do not allow it to become clogged with too much detail. Layout ideas can be gleaned by looking through newspapers and magazines or, better still, from graphic design books and journals. If possible, discuss these ideas with a graphic artist. The layout should be clear, logical and suitable for the material being presented. Try a number of different rough layouts first and seek the opinion of a colleague to determine the best. A possible layout is shown in Figure 4.2.

Plan to mount components onto panels of coloured card cut to sizes convenient to transport. An alternative is to get the whole poster photographically enlarged to full size. It can be carried rolled up in a cardboard or plastic tube.

FIGURE 4.2.
POSSIBLE LAYOUT FOR A
CONFERENCE POSTER

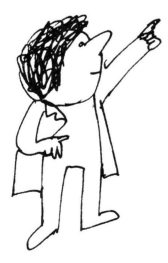

Text should be large enough to be read at the viewing distance, which is likely to be about one metre. In this case, we suggest that the smallest letters be at least 5 mm high and preferably larger. Good quality titles and text can be produced with a word-processor and a high-resolution printer. These can be enlarged, as required, photographically or on a photocopier. Consider using colour to highlight specific points.

Break up the density of text into several discrete parts. For example, consider dividing the text into an abstract, an introduction, a statement of method, results and conclusion each with its own clear heading. A short list of references or of publications arising out of your work might also be appropriate.

Remember, that in preparing your poster you are really trying to achieve many of the same things you would wish to achieve with a talk or lecture: attract interest and generally communicate effectively.

CHAIRING A CONFERENCE SESSION

Much of the success of a conference will depend on the quality of the chairing of individual sessions. Should this task fall to you, there are many responsibilities to fulfil. There are three categories of tasks – responsibilities to the organisers, to the speaker and to the audience.

Responsibilities to the organisers

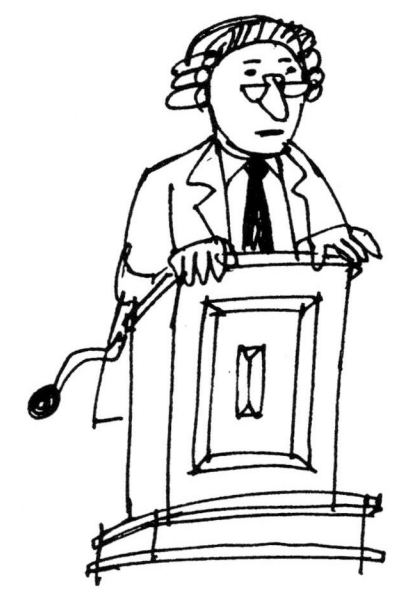

The organisers of the conference will have approached you several months before the event. If you are lucky, they will also have given you detailed guidelines to follow but if not you must, at a minimum, find out:

★ The time and length of the session.
★ The number and names of the speakers.
★ A copy of the instructions given to speakers with particular reference to the time allocated for the presentation and the time allocated for discussion.
★ Whether there are concurrent sessions.

Ideally you will contact the speakers in advance of the conference to ensure they have indeed received instructions and understand their implication, particularly with regard to time. You may find that some are inexperienced and nervous about the prospect of their presentation and your advice will be appreciated. Referring the speaker to the earliest parts of this chapter might be valuable.

If early contact has not been made, it is essential to meet with speakers prior to the session. You must clarify the format of the session and reinforce your intention to stick rigidly to the allocated time. You should explain the method to be used to indicate when there is one minute to go, when time is up and what steps you will take should the speaker continue for longer. This may sound draconian but, believe us, it is vital. A timing device on the lectern is an invaluable aid to compliance.

Prior to the session, you must also familiarise yourself with the layout of the venue, the audio-visual facilities and the lighting. In the absence of a technician, you may be called on to operate the equipment and lighting or to instruct the speakers in their use.

At the start of the session, announce that you intend to keep to time and do so.

Finally, you must be certain that the session and individual presentations commence and finish at the programmed time. This is particularly important when there are concurrent sessions.

Responsibilities to the speakers

Speakers invariably fall into one of three types.

The well-organised speakers: they will tell you exactly what they are going to do and what they require. If you ask them how long they are going to speak, they will tell you in minutes and seconds! You will need to have little concern for these speakers, but they will expect you be as well prepared and organised as themselves.

The apprehensive speakers: they will generally be the younger and less experienced. They will often have a well-prepared paper to present but are in danger of not doing themselves justice. You can assist such speakers greatly by familiarising them with the facilities before the session and encouraging them to practise operating the audio-visual equipment. If this seems beyond them, you may be able to take on this task yourself. Calm reassurance that all will be well is the message to convey.

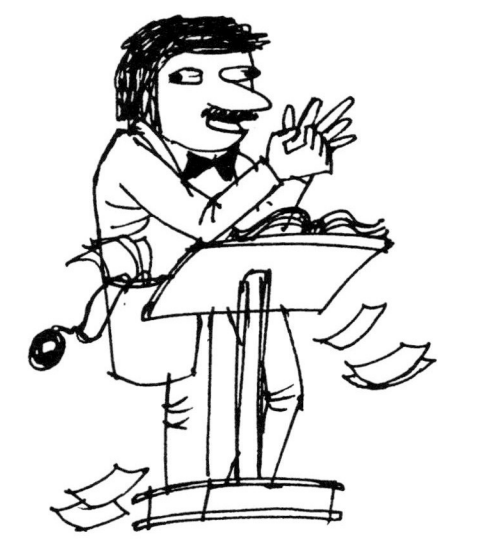

The confident under-prepared speakers: these are remarkably prevalent and the most dangerous for the chairperson. They will not seek advice and will deny having received detailed instructions about their presentation. When you ask them how long they expect to speak, you will receive an off-hand response. They will tell you that they have not rehearsed their presentation and will almost certainly go over time. There is little you can do to help such people because they are certain they have everything under control. However, they can be your downfall unless you prepare to intervene. Prior to the session you must convince them you are serious about cutting them off if they speak over time. Unfortunately this strategy will often fail and you must be prepared to act immediately the first time a speaker goes over the allotted time. After a maximum of 15 seconds grace, rise from your chair. If the hint is not immediately taken, you have no option but to politely but firmly stop the speaker. Examples can be cited of such speakers being physically led off the stage still talking, but such extremes should not arise. Fortunately, you will only have to intervene in such a way once in a session and, should it happen, your future as an invited chairperson is assured.

In the discussion period you must see fair play. Ensure that questions are relevant and brief. Do not allow a questioner to make long statements or commence a mini-presentation of their own work. Suggest any significant differences of opinion be explored informally at the subsequent coffee break.

Responsibilities to the audience

The audience has a right to expect several things. They must be able to hear the speaker and see the slides. They must be reassured that you will keep the speakers to time to protect their opportunity to ask questions and to allow them to move to any concurrent sessions. Speakers going over time is the commonest complaint of participants and the chair is usually held to blame. During the question period you should ensure that the time is not monopolised by the intellectual heavies in the front rows. On the other hand you must also be prepared to ask the first question if none is immediately forthcoming from the audience.

Finishing off

At the close of the session, thank the speakers and the audience and remind them of the starting time of the next session. You may also have been asked to transmit information from the organisers. Particularly important would be to obtain completed evaluation forms for the session if these had been provided.

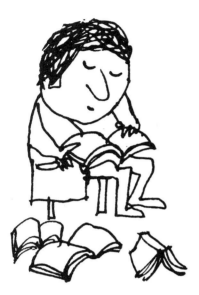

GUIDED READING

The book we can still recommend for further reading is J. Calnan and A. Barabas' *Speaking at Medical Meetings*, Heinemann, London, 1981. This pocket-sized do-it-yourself guide is not only valuable but also entertaining. It contains many useful illustrations and good advice about the preparation of visual aids.

Another manual is P. Race's *Conference Presentations and Workshops*, University of Northumbria, 1986 (available through Amazon.co.uk).

Those interested in the organisation and evaluation of medical meetings are referred to a series entitled *Improving Medical Meetings*, written by D. Richmond and his colleagues, published in the *British Medical Journal* (1983), **287**, pp. 1201-2; 1286-7; 1363-4; 1450-1.

For help with the design of charts and graphs check the references at the end of Chapter 9.

An excellent general text on public speaking is C. Turk's *Effective Speaking*, Spon, London, 1985. This is a comprehensive reference work that has been written by a university lecturer.

Another comprehensive resource is S. Lucas' *The Art of Public Speaking*, McGraw Hill, 2000.

5: TEACHING PRACTICAL AND CLINICAL SKILLS

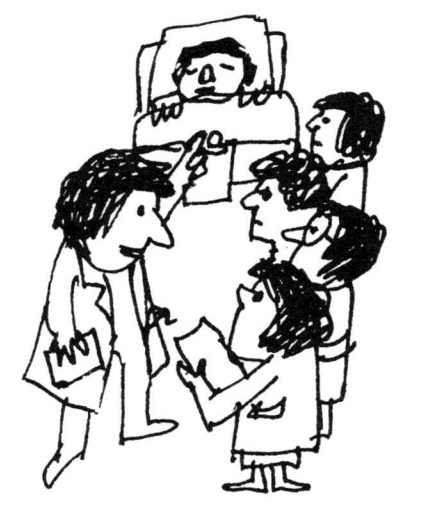

INTRODUCTION

In the first part of this chapter we plan to look at ways of improving your clinical teaching. Later in the chapter we will address the issue of practical and laboratory based teaching.

While it is increasingly likely that your institution will provide some form of 'teach the teachers' course it is relatively unlikely that it will specifically address clinical teaching. It is a fact that clinical teaching is the most neglected area of all teaching despite being the one where more deficiencies have been found than in any other. The conclusion of one extensive study was that 'many (clinical) teaching sessions, particularly ward rounds, were haphazard, mediocre and lacking in intellectual excitement'. In one study of medical schools in North America, it was stated that there were few students who could report having been monitored in the interview and physical examination of more than one or two patients and that a surprising number had been awarded their degree without ever having been properly supervised in the complete data-collecting process of even one patient! It is our experience, with notable exceptions, that a similar situation can be found in many medical schools in other parts of the world.

THE ATTRIBUTES OF AN EFFECTIVE CLINICAL TEACHER

These have been identified on the basis of the opinions of experts, the perceptions of students and from the observations of actual clinical teaching. Considering the limited nature of the research there is a remarkable consistency in the results. It might be helpful to start by checking yourself against these attributes.

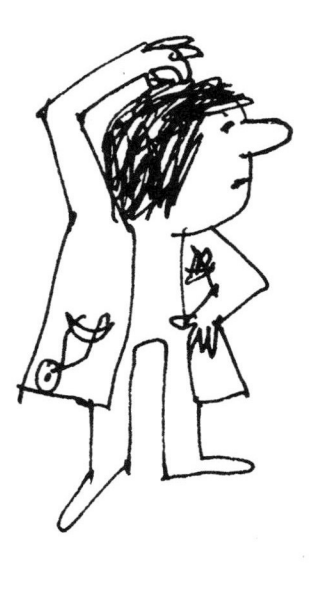

★ Do you encourage active participation by the students and avoid having them stand around in an observational capacity?

★ Do you have and demonstrate a positive attitude to your teaching?

★ Is the emphasis of your teaching on applied problem solving?

★ Do you focus on the integration of clinical medicine with the basic and clinical sciences or do you spend most of the time on didactic teaching of factual material?

★ Do you closely supervise the students as they interview and examine patients at the bedside and provide effective feedback on their performance or do you rely on their verbal case presentations in the teaching room?

★ Do you provide adequate opportunities for your students to practice their skills?

★ Do you provide a good role model, particularly in the area of interpersonal relationships with your patients?

★ Does your teaching provide stimulation and challenge?

★ Is your teaching generally patient-orientated or does it tend to be disease-orientated?

★ Are you friendly, helpful and available to your students?

Should your honest answer to some of these questions be 'no' then you are probably a typical clinical teacher as many studies have shown that all of these characteristics are rarely present. Just becoming aware of such attributes should encourage you to be more critical of your approach. The remainder of this chapter will deal more specifically with the planning and the techniques which can be introduced to enhance the effectiveness of your clinical teaching.

IMPROVING CLINICAL TEACHING

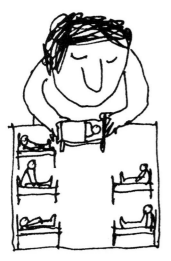

If you are a clinical teacher with no responsibilities for the planning of the curriculum, there may be few educational initiatives open to you other than to improve your hospital-based or community-based teaching. What you should aim to do is to try and acquire as many as possible of the attributes described in the previous section. There are no hard and fast rules as to how you can achieve this aim but the following points may be helpful.

Plan the teaching: it is possible that you will have received highly specific instructions from the medical school particularly if you are teaching in a structured programme (see later). If not, it is worthwhile contacting the department head or the course co-ordinator to see if there are defined objectives for the part of the curriculum in which your teaching is placed.

If these are not forthcoming, you should draw up your own objectives, at least to the extent of writing down what you hope to achieve during the students' attachment. In doing so you must taken into account your time, the duration of the students' attachment, the number of students and the seniority of the students. You must be realistic about what you can achieve and not attempt to cram too much into your sessions. You should inform the students about the plan when they start and listen to any comments they may make which might reasonably give you cause to modify the plan. Though clinical teaching is essentially opportunistic, being dependent on the availability of patients, it is wise to keep a record of the conditions seen during your teaching so that by the end of the course you have covered a wide enough range of illustrative cases. You should, of course, co-ordinate your teaching with other tutors who are involved with your group of students.

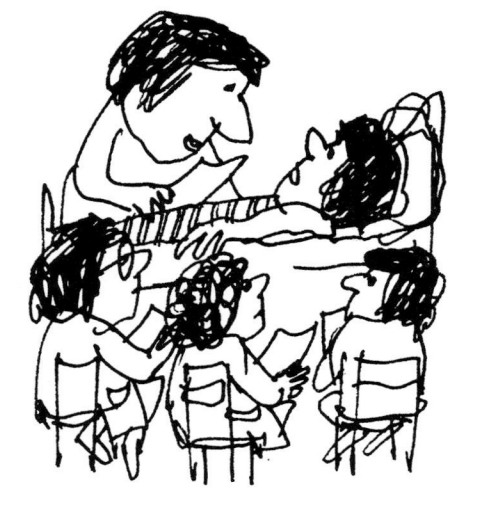

Set a good example: it is surprising how infrequently students get the chance to watch an experienced clinician take a history, perform an examination and subsequently discuss the outcome and plans with the patient. It is normally impossible to do this on a working hospital ward round because pressure of time means that decision-making is given priority. However, the outpatient department or a community practice setting often provide better opportunities.

One of the difficulties students might have under such circumstances is the contrast between what you do in practice and what you expect of the students. This issue may have to be discussed. The important thing is for the students to see you in action, particularly in regard to the way you relate to the patients while at the same time achieve the medical aims of the encounter. Even in busy clinical situations it is important to demonstrate a concern for the patient's feelings.

Involve the student: the need for active participation is the recurrent theme throughout this book and nowhere is it more important than in the clinical teaching situation. You should take every opportunity to ask students to perform. This may range from talking to a patient, checking physical signs, presenting the case history, answering questions and looking up clinical information for presentation at the next teaching session. In general try and make sure all the tasks are directly related to the patients the student has seen. The emphasis of the teaching should be 'bedside not backside'.

Observe the student: as mentioned earlier, a consistent finding in studies of clinical teaching has been a lack of direct observation of student interactions with patients. All too often the clinical teacher starts with the case presentation and many never check to see whether the features described are actually present or were elicited personally by the student. Serious deficiencies in clinical skills are consistently found in interns and residents which must be an indictment of the undergraduate clinical teaching. Only a commitment to the somewhat boring task of observing the student take the history, perform the physical examination and explain things to the patient will allow you to identify and correct any deficiencies. This type of activity is particularly essential with junior students and must be conducted in a sympathetic and supportive way.

Provide a good teaching environment: the more senior and prestigious you are, the more intimidating you are likely to appear to the students. It is vital that you adopt a friendly and helpful manner and reduce the natural and inevitable apprehension felt by your students. Not only may they be apprehensive about you, but they will also be apprehensive about their impending contact with patients. You can assist this by preparing the patients and by showing to the students you understand their fears. Such fears are likely to be particularly evident with junior students.

IMPROVING THE CLINICAL TUTORIAL

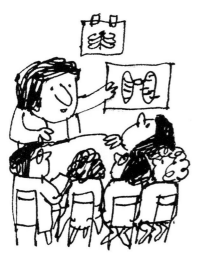

Clinical tutorials are all too often didactic with the emphasis being on a disease rather than on the solving of patient problems. We firmly believe the clinical teacher should concentrate on the latter. The students will inevitably have many other opportunities to acquire factual information but relatively little time to grapple with the more difficult task of learning to apply their knowledge to patient problems. It is sad, but true, that in traditional medical schools the students are often as much to blame as their teachers by encouraging didactic presentations, particularly when examinations are imminent. Surprisingly, clinical teaching in problem-based schools often exhibits the same characteristics.

Plan the teaching: once again it is important to establish the aims of the sessions you have been allocated. There may be fixed topics to cover or you may have a free hand. In either case you must be sure in your own mind what you intend to achieve in each session.

Involve the student: make it clear from the beginning that you expect most of the talking to be done by the students and that all of them are to participate, not just the vocal minority. At the first session, explain what tasks you expect them to perform in preparation for each tutorial. You may, for example, expect them to prepare cases for discussion or to read up aspects of the literature on a particular subject.

Provide a good teaching environment: the way in which you set up the session is vital for its success, particularly when you wish to encourage active participation. Your role as a facilitator, not the fount of all knowledge, must be emphasised and you must resist the temptation to intervene with extra information all the time. This is very hard to avoid but if it happens too frequently you will soon find all conversation is channelled in your direction and there will be no interaction between the students.

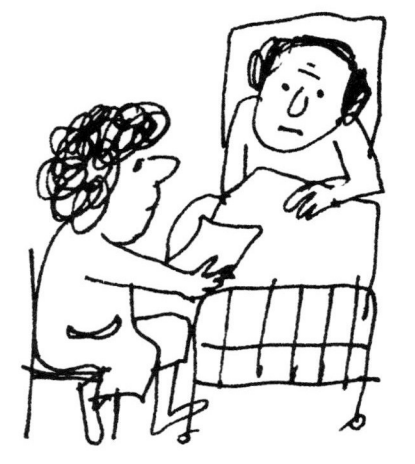

As the clinical tutorial is another form of small group teaching you should read Chapter 4 for further advice.

Concentrate on clinical problem solving: in the last thirty years there has been a substantial research effort into how doctors and students go about solving clinical problems. The findings have major implications for the clinical teacher, though as yet there is little evidence that this has been widely recognised. The traditional way of teaching students is to require them to take a full history, perform a comprehensive examination and only then come up with a differential diagnosis. The implication has been that clinical examination is a routine and sequential process with serious thinking about diagnosis and management being deferred until the student is away from the bedside. This is not the way doctors or students actually operate even though they may appear to do so on superficial observation.

Research has shown that experienced clinicians will generate diagnostic hypotheses within a minute or so of first seeing the patient. The bulk of time spent interviewing and examining the patient will then be used to confirm or refute these hypotheses. This approach to problem solving is a natural ability and does not have to be taught in its own right. However, successful clinical problem solving is dependent on previous experience with similar problems and on effective utilisation of the person's medical knowledge base relevant to the problem. These findings provide one of the arguments for why increasing numbers of medical schools are using problem-based learning as the keystone of the curriculum. Patient problems are used to trigger the search for factual information rather than teaching factual information before exposing students to patient problems (see Chapter 7).

How to teach clinical problem solving: from what we have said the aim must be to provide your students with as much experience as possible in manipulating their factual knowledge in relation to patient problems. You should avoid conducting tutorials in which you or your students simply present topics. If, for example, you wish to have a tutorial dealing with hypertension then a patient with hypertension should be the focus. The student will then be required to consider the implications of hypertension in relation to that particular patient. Figure 5.1 briefly shows a plan for the simplest type of problem solving tutorial.

FIGURE 5.1.
A PLAN FOR A PROBLEM-
SOLVING TUTORIAL

Procedure

- A week before the tutorial, designate one or two students to prepare a case for presentation. Tell them they are to be prepared on all clinical and theoretical aspects of the case.
- At the start of the tutorial outline the aims of the exercise.
- Get the prepared students to give the presenting complaint or allow the patient to tell the story.
- Stop, and ask the other students what they think the problem or diagnosis could be. Ask them to justify their suggestions. Encourage the other students to react to these suggestions.
- Allow the presentation of more data.
- Stop again, and ask the group whether they have changed their views and why.
- Continue the process.

This general approach is used not just for data gathering but also for the ordering of investigations (what tests would you order and why?) and treatment (what treatment would you give and why?). Though this may sound rather structured and formal, in practice this will not be so. You will soon learn to judge the pace, learn how much new information is to be given before stopping and so on. However, you may initially find sessions of this type hard going if the students are not used to the challenge of this method of teaching. Those previously relying on the regurgitation of lists and pages from the books may be particularly discomforted. They may attempt to avoid answering or justifying their suggestions but persistence will pay off.

With sessions of this type it is important to create a non-threatening atmosphere. One way of helping is to participate yourself. Let the presenting students bring along a case or patient whom you do not know. Still encourage the students to answer first but you can then add your own thoughts. You may even find this more threatening than the students but it is important they learn that infallibility is not an attribute of clinical teachers and that it is quite normal for even the most experienced clinician to have to admit indecision and a need to obtain advice or further information.

ALTERNATIVES TO TRADITIONAL CLINICAL TEACHING

We have already provided evidence that traditional clinical teaching is often inadequate in meeting the aims of both the medical school and the students. This has led many schools to introduce structured courses to teach basic clinical skills in a less haphazard manner. The skills taught are often not restricted to interviewing and physical examination but include technical skills and clinical problem solving. Should you have the opportunity to introduce or participate in such an approach then the first step must be to define the objectives of the exercise. These must take into account the seniority of the students, the time allocated in the curriculum, the facilities, and the availability of teachers and other resources. There are obviously many ways in which this could be done but we will restrict ourselves to outlining such a programme

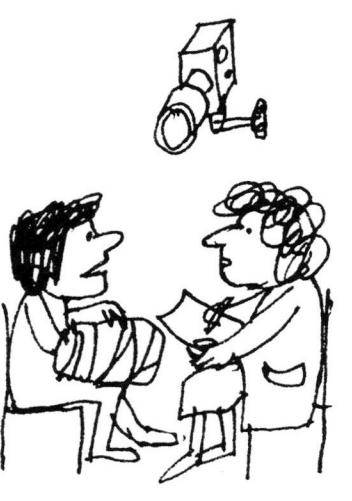

which has been run successfully for many years jointly by a Department of Medicine and a Department of Surgery. It is one which has retained the support of both staff and students.

The course plan for the programme is shown in Figure 5.2. In the left-land column you can see the objectives. Opposite each are the teaching activities which are planned to help the student achieve the objectives. In the right-hand column are the assessment procedures which are also matched to the objectives. You can see that a range of methods is used. The key to the programme is the attachment of only three students to a preceptor for instruction on history taking and physical examination. You will note that the problem-orientated medical record approach has been adopted and we find this has been a valuable adjunct to our teaching. Whole-group problem-solving sessions include clinical decision making, emergency care, data interpretation (clinical chemistry, haematology and imaging) and management/therapeutics. The students are also expected to take responsibility for a lot of their own learning.

FIGURE 5.2.
PLAN FOR A STRUCTURED COURSE ON BASIC CLINICAL SKILLS

OBJECTIVES	TEACHING ACTIVITIES	ASSESSMENT
TAKE A COMPREHENSIVE HISTORY	PRECEPTOR SESSIONS WITH VIDEO RECORDINGS. WARD ACTIVITIES	PRECEPTOR'S JUDGEMENT BASED ON REPEAT OBSERVATIONS
PERFORM A COMPLETE PHYSICAL EXAMINATION	VIEWING DEMONSTRATION VIDEO. PRECEPTOR SESSIONS. WARD PRACTICE. WARD ROUNDS WITH REGISTRARS	PRECEPTOR'S JUDGEMENT. OBSERVATION OF COMPLETE PHYSICAL EXAMINATION BY INDEPENDENT EXAMINER AT END OF COURSE
WRITE-UP HISTORY AND EXAMINATION AND CONSTRUCT A PROBLEM LIST	PROBLEM-ORIENTED CASE WRITE-UPS ON WARD PATIENTS. PRECEPTOR SESSIONS	CASE WRITE-UPS
DECISIONS ON DIAGNOSIS, INVESTIGATIONS AND MANAGEMENT	WHOLE-GROUP PROBLEM-SOLVING SESSIONS. CASE WRITE-UPS	WHOLE GROUP TUTOR'S OPINION. CASE WRITE-UPS
ABILITY TO RELATE TO PATIENTS	PRECEPTOR SESSIONS WITH REVIEW OF VIDEO RECORDINGS	PRECEPTOR'S JUDGEMENT
IMPROVE KNOWLEDGE OF MEDICINE AND SURGERY	SELF-INSTRUCTION. PREPARATION OF CASES FOR PRESENTATION TO THE WHOLE GROUP. COMPUTERIZED SELF-ASSESS-MENT PROGRAMMES. TAPE–SLIDE TUTORIALS	WHOLE-GROUP TUTOR'S OPINION. SELF-ASSESSMENT

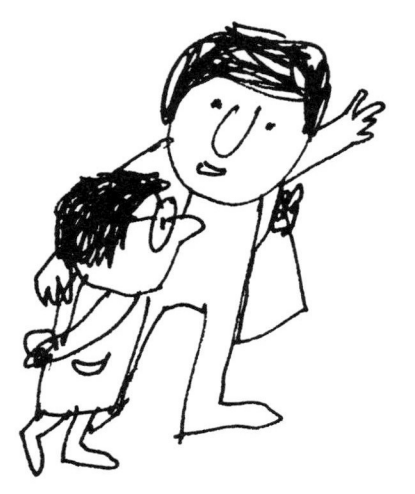

As it has been decided that the time of the teaching staff should be devoted to preceptoring and conducting small group sessions, the revision of the theoretical aspects of medicine and surgery is left entirely to the students. Various self-learning materials are also available for the students to use in their own time.

Though such a programme is far from perfect, it was introduced within a traditional curriculum and with the minimum of resources. The main change was a reallocation of staff time away from didactic activities and into more direct observation of student performance.

A perusal of the medical educational literature will provide you with other examples of structured clinical teaching. Increasingly you will find descriptions of the use of **clinical skills laboratories** where medical schools have set up fully staffed and equipped areas devoted to putting groups of students through an intensive training in clinical skills, often using a wide range of simulations. You will also find many examples of training students in interpersonal and communication skills using simulated patients. All have the same general approach: to undertake the training of various clinical skills in a structured and supervised way to ensure that all students achieve a basic level of competence.

TECHNIQUES FOR TEACHING PARTICULAR PRACTICAL AND CLINICAL SKILLS

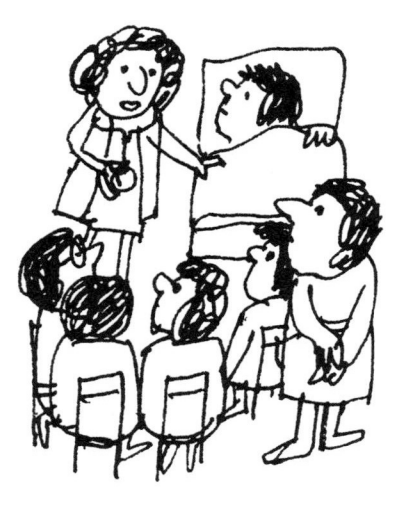

Many practical and clinical skills can be taught as separate elements. Because there is a wide range of these elements, and as clinical teaching is generally opportunistic, many medical schools have established programmes to teach basic skills in a piecemeal fashion. This is normally done early in the students' career, often just prior to their first clinical attachments. Much of this has come about because of new technology (e.g. video recording, computers) and because of an awareness of the value of simulation in its many forms. This section will introduce you to a variety of ways of teaching basic skills some of which may not be of immediate relevance but some of which ought to be in operation in your medical school because of their proven efficacy.

The clinical interview

There are two basic methods with which you should be familiar; the use of video recordings and the use of simulation.

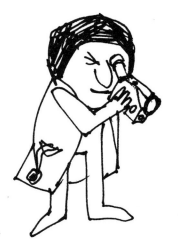

Video recording: any department which has the responsibility for teaching aspects of history taking or inter-personal skills should have access to video recording equipment, preferably of the portable kind that can be set up in ward side rooms, outpatients and other teaching situations. You should become familiar with the technical operation of the equipment.

There are several ways in which video equipment can be used. The simplest is to record examples of interviewing techniques (good and bad) for demonstration purposes. This may be valuable as a starting point for new students. You may also wish to have an example of a basic general history so the novice student can get an idea of the questions that are routinely asked. Some medical schools have recorded segments of interviews with patients which show various emotional reactions (e.g. aggressive beha-viour, grief, manipulation).

The most powerful way of using the video is to record the student's interview with a patient remembering that informed consent is essential. This may be initially stressful but both student and patient usually forget they are being recorded after a few minutes. A time limit of 20-30 minutes is advisable. The student, or a small group of students, meet later with the teacher to review the tape. It is at this stage that some skill by the teacher is required. Firstly, the situation must be a supportive one to allow frank and open discussion. Secondly, the teacher must have a clear idea of what the students should be learning. (If you have not read formally in the area of the clinical interview, we would recommend the book by Cole and Bird.)

It is not appropriate to play the tape completely through and then have a discussion. The tape must be stopped frequently to discuss points as they arise. Such things as non-verbal cues, aspects of doctor-patient relationships, avoidance of jargon, adequacy of questions, direction of the enquiry, directive versus non-directive questioning, hypothesis generation and many other issues can be

81

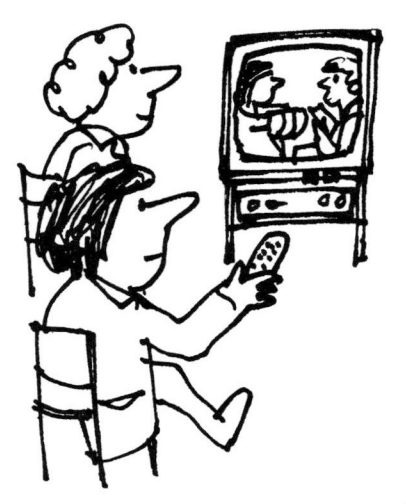

identified and discussed, both with the interviewing student and with the student's peers. Such sessions are valuable both with junior and senior students.

There are clearly several advantages of this approach over direct observation: the teacher is not committed to be present at the actual interview; the teaching can be scheduled at a convenient time; a recorded interview can be interrupted as often as necessary; and most importantly the students can review their own performance. The latter by itself often produces a striking impact and a rapid improvement in competence.

Simulation: the use of simulated (or standardised) patients is another well-proven and powerful method for teaching interview skills. However, if does require some expertise to train the simulated patients and if you wish to pursue this technique we strongly recommend that you read the book by Barrows. The simulated patient offers certain distinct advantages over the real patient particularly for the novice student. The analogy has been drawn with the value of flight deck simulators in pilot training. The advantages include: the ability to schedule interviews at a convenient time and place; all students can be faced with the same situation; the interview can be interrupted and any problems discussed freely in front of the 'patient'; there is no risk of offending or harming the patient (often a concern of new students); the student can take as much time as necessary; the same 'patient' can be re-interviewed at a later date; and the simulator can be trained to provide direct feedback, particularly in the area of doctor-patient relationships.

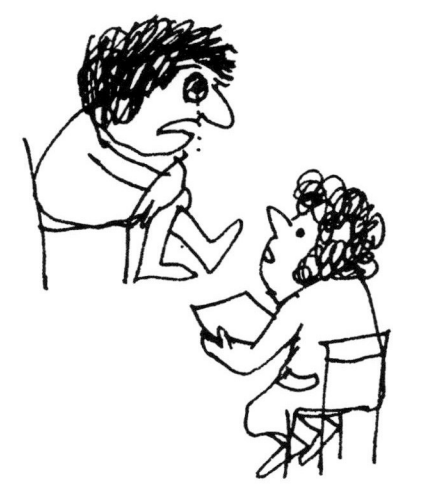

Simulations can also be developed for situations that are usually impossible for students to experience with real patients. This is particularly so for emotionally charged areas. With all these advantages it is surprising how long it has taken for this technique to become widely used. Much is due to uninformed prejudice. Some is due to a lack of appreciation as to how easy it is to train simulated patients. This is not an appropriate place to deal with this aspect in depth. However, it is important to remember that it is not essential to use actors. In fact our preference is to avoid actors, who may wish to give a performance rather than be a 'patient'. The basic technique is to identify a patient with the condition you wish to simulate. A protocol is drawn up of the facts which are relevant to that condition. All other aspects of this history not relevant to the condition need not be simulated, i.e. the simulator's own background can be used or adapted. The simulator then learns the role, including non-verbal cues. The trainer then tests the simulation by taking the history. Modifications are made and further practice sessions conducted. It is then our practice to try out the simulation, for example, by asking one of the resident staff to conduct an interview. This is observed and a discussion held with the resident about the patient. It is readily apparent whether the resident suspects the simulator of not being real. It is, in fact, vary rare for a well-trained simulator to be suspected, which is a good confidence booster for both the simulator and trainer.

The physical examination

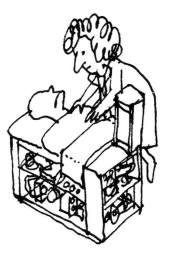

Video recording: video recordings can be used to help students develop physical examination skills in much the same way as for interviewing skills. However, it is not quite so effective and direct observation and instruction are generally more appropriate. It is very valuable to have videos which illustrate the recommended way of performing specific components of the examination. These must be readily available to students together with convenient playback facilities.

Simulation devices: this is the area where technology has made a major contribution. The number of these devices is increasing rapidly and includes those for cardiac auscultation, breast examination, prostate palpatation, pelvic examination and laryngeal examination. They are often to be found in skills laboratories.

Simulated patients: these can also be used in very much the same way as for history taking, with similar advantages. However, the range of signs that can be simulated is limited, though not as much as you might think. For example, Barrows in his classic book showed that a wide range of neurological conditions can be simulated.

In regard to other systems, conditions where pain is the main feature are particularly suitable. Also valuable are simulations of emergency situations such as perforation of a viscus, myocardial infarction and subarachnoid haemorrhage. Students can be trained to perform rapid assessment and acute management for conditions that otherwise would be impossible to programme.

Simulated patient instructors are widely used, particularly in North America, to teach the pelvic examination. The main advantage of such an approach is that the instructor gives direct feedback on the students' performance. The instructor is the only one who can say if the student has correctly palpated the ovaries and uterus or whether unnecessary discomfort has been created. The same approach has been used to teach rectal examinations in the male.

Though not simulation, it is perhaps worthwhile remembering that self and peer examination is a valuable teaching technique for novice students. The learning of many basic manual skills is much better done in this way than using real patients.

The use of instruments and basic equipment

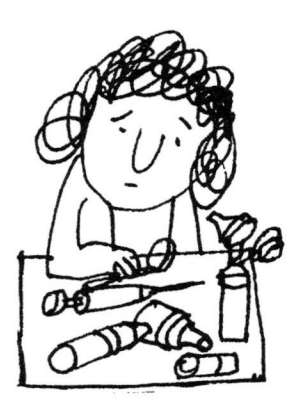

The student has to become competent with a variety of instruments and basic medical equipment other than the stethoscope. These include the opthalmoscope, the auroscope, the proctoscope, the laryngoscope, syringes, infusion apparatus, and endotracheal tubes. For many of these, simulation devices are available. In most cases it is inappropriate for the first attempt to use them to be made on a patient. Students certainly appreciate the chance to practice their skills in a situation where they are not going to hurt a patient.

Some techniques, of course, are readily practiced on each other (e.g. examinations of the eyes, ears and throat).

TEACHING PRACTICAL AND LABORATORY CLASSES

Practical and laboratory classes are often regarded as an essential component of science-based courses. However, they are becoming less prevalent in the medical curriculum as the pressures to free up time for other components in the course and decreasing resources force a re-appraisal of their value. We have decided not to give detailed consideration to these important areas of teaching in this book but to refer those with responsibilities of this type to more specific resources. These are listed at the end of this chapter and include the non-medical version of our book entitled ''A Handbook for Teachers in Universities and Colleges''. However, there is one particular type of practical teaching that we will mention, that is the research project, which is equally as likely to be managed by clinical teachers as by basic science teachers.

Research projects

Research projects have always held an important place in science-based courses. There is now a growing appreciation of their value, albeit in a more limited and less technically demanding form, at various phases of the medical curriculum. Projects should provide the student with a real-life experience of research that is quite different to the more controlled laboratory exercises. They are strongly motivational to most students because of the high level of active participation, the close contact with supervisors and research staff, the lower emphasis on assessment and the greater degree of personal responsibility.

Research projects can be undertaken individually, by groups, or by attachment to a research team in which the student accepts responsibility for certain aspects of an established project. Whatever the approach, the role of the supervisor is critical. Should this be your role, the points outlined in Figure 5.3 should be remembered.

FIGURE 5.3.
TASKS FOR THE SUPERVISOR
OF A RESEARCH PROJECT

Procedure

- Meet with the student and agree on the objectives of the exercise and the problem to be researched.
- Work out a schedule of work covering the period during which the project is to be conducted, with provisional deadlines for completion of each stage (e.g. literature review, hypothesis generation and experimental design; experimental work; data analysis; report).
- Arrange a regular meeting time with students to check progress (remember the task is to guide not direct).
- Assist the student to prepare the final report or to give the seminar presentation by means of critical discussion and practice (Students could be referred to the appropriate sections in this book!).

Supervisors vary markedly in their commitment and skill. It is recommended that departments using research projects should provide guidelines and training for supervisors. Most institutions now run courses and provide suitable handbooks. Several valuable publications are available that could be used or modified for this purpose (see Guided Reading at the end of this chapter).

Alternative methods

A combination of modern technology and interest in new teaching techniques has provided alternatives to the conventional approaches to practical work. Two that are now well established are computer-based methods and simulations.

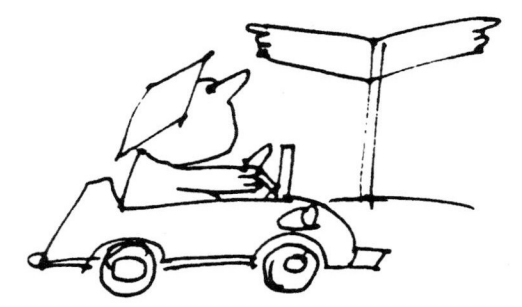

Computer-based methods

The wide availability of computers and their everyday use in all areas of science and technology makes their integration into practical courses almost essential. Early in the curriculum, there may be a need to have practical classes to teach students how to use computers.

In the laboratory setting, computers may be interfaced with other equipment or used to enhance or even replace conventional practical work.

Learning the skills of data analysis and interpretation is often linked to laboratory teaching. With the computer, it is possible to provide students with a wide range of data sets on which they can practice these skills at varying levels of complexity and sophistication.

Simulations

Simulations are playing an increasingly important role in practical teaching for many reasons. Some reflect a need to provide repetitive practice of basic and advanced skills which might not otherwise be readily available, be too complex (e.g. acquiring of experimental data) or too dangerous (e.g. trainee medical staff performing operative procedures). The types of simulations also vary widely, ranging from simple drill and practice (e.g. using equipment; taking blood samples) through to replacing the need for live animal experiments. The computer is, of course, involved in many of the more complex simulations. The increasing sophistication of graphics and virtual reality will ensure a burgeoning industry in the instructional application of computer-based simulations.

EVALUATING CLINICAL AND PRACTICAL TEACHING

There are few well-developed procedures for evaluating your performance as a clinical teacher. The major reason for this is that much clinical teaching is done on a one-to-one basis or in very small groups over relatively short periods of time. This causes a problem in obtaining valid and reliable information about performance. However, this deficiency is a matter of concern and research is underway to develop more useful instruments. You can, of course, adapt the principles and procedures described in the chapter on small group teaching and integrate these with the checklist displayed at the very beginning of this chapter.

You may have gained the impression that we favour the exclusive use of questionnaires in evaluation. We wish to point out that this is not the case. Questionnaires are only one method which seek data from one source – typically your students. In all evaluation, including clinical and practical teaching, we would wish to encourage you to explore other methods and other sources of evaluative information which you will encounter throughout this book.

GUIDED READING

Although there are many good books written on how to perform a medical interview and a physical examination, there seems to be a dearth of recent books on clinical teaching.

The Physician as Teacher by T. Schwenk and N. Whitman, Williams & Wilkins, Baltimore, 1987, is still a useful guide to the tasks faced by a medical teacher, including clinical teaching.

A useful recent resource is a series of articles representing the output of the Ninth Cambridge Conference on Medical

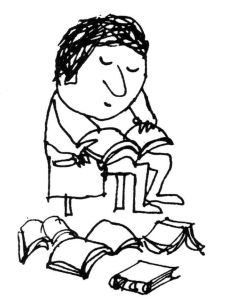

Education which appear in *Medical Education* (2000), **34**, No 10. The topic of this conference was *Clinical Teaching and its Assessment*.

For additional information on practical and laboratory teaching we recommend the following:

A Handbook for Teaching and Learning in Universities and Colleges by R. Cannon and D. Newble, Kogan Page, London, 2000.

Improving Teaching and Learning in Laboratories by E. Hazel and C. Baillie, HERDSA Gold Guide No 4, 1998 available from HERDSA, PO Box 51, Jamieson, ACT, 2614, Australia.

Teaching in Laboratories by D. Boud, J. Dunn and E. Hegarty-Hazel, Open University Press, Guildford, 1989.

Books and articles referred to in this chapter:

S. Cole and J. Bird. *The Medical Interview*. Mosby Year Book, 1999.

H. Barrows. *Simulated Patients (Programmed Patients)*. Charles C. Thomas, Springfield, 1971.

6: PLANNING A COURSE

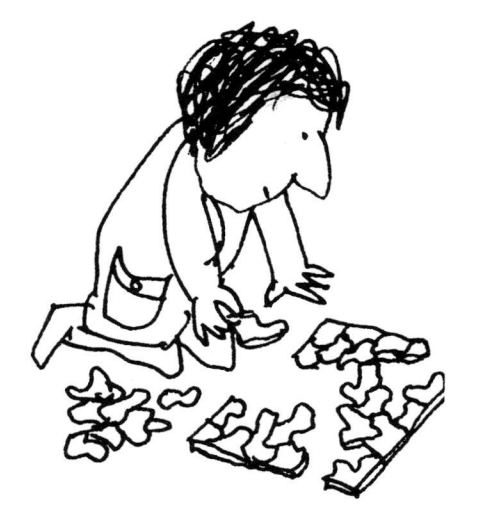

INTRODUCTION

This chapter aims to assist you when you become involved in some way in curriculum planning and wish to do so in a systematic manner. Unfortunately, there is no straightforward formula to guide you in this activity. The reasons for this are as follows. First, curriculum planning is a complex business involving more than purely educational considerations. For example, you will find that full account must be taken of the political and economic context in which you teach. Second, relatively few courses are started from scratch. Much curriculum development is a matter of revising and adapting existing courses or materials. And third, there are important differences between individuals – especially between individuals working in different disciplines – in the ways in which they view a variety of educational issues. You may, for instance, see your main function as transmitting appropriate knowledge, skills and attitudes. On the other hand you may perceive your role as being primarily concerned with the personal and social development of your students as well as with their intellectual development. In a book of this kind it is not possible to provide a discussion which can fully take into account these various orientations. However, we believe that you should be aware of these differences and we would encourage you to read further on the matter to help develop your own particular orientation and your own approach to curriculum development.

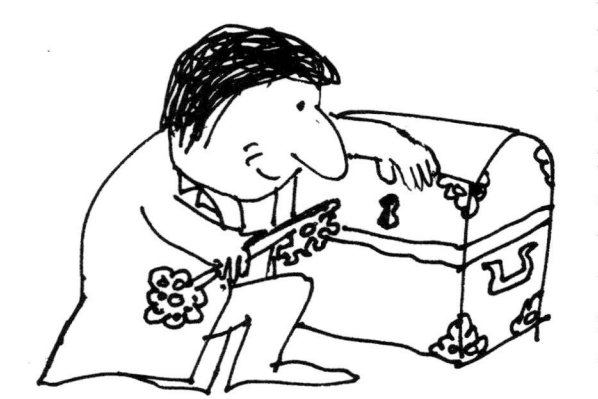

In our view, the key to good curriculum or course design is to forge educationally sound and logical links between planned intentions (expressed as objectives), course content, teaching and learning methods, and the assessment of student learning while taking account of student characteristics. In the past, too many courses started with vague intentions, consisted of teaching which had a tenuous relationship to these intentions and employed methods of assessment which bore little or no relationship to either. Such courses then placed students in the unfortunate situation of playing a guessing game, with their academic future as the stake! This pattern can be improved by adopting an approach which aligns the intentions with course content, teaching, and the assessment.

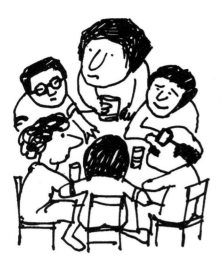

WHO SHOULD BE RESPONSIBLE FOR CURRICULUM PLANNING?

Although we assume you have some responsibility for course planning, it is unlikely that this will be a solo affair. You will have additional resources on which to draw which may include colleagues in your own and related departments, staff of a university teaching unit, members of your discipline outside your immediate environment, and students. These people may form a planning committee or a panel of advisers. Whatever your situation, experience suggests that some form of consultation with others is very desirable.

COURSE CONTENT

Content is a broad concept meant to include all aspects of knowledge, skills and attitudes relevant to the course and to the intellectual experiences of students and their teachers in a course.

While not always easy to achieve, we feel that course content should be made explicit and that this will then put you in a better position to make informed and coherent decisions in your planning. There are several different criteria for selecting content that may be more or less relevant to your work. These criteria are presented below for your consideration.

Academic criteria

These criteria focus attention on theoretical, methodological and value positions. For example:

- Content should be a means of enhancing the intellectual development of students, not an end in itself.
- Content that is solely concerned with technical matters has a limited place in university education; content must also involve moral and ethical considerations.
- Content should contribute to a deep rather than to a surface view of knowledge.

Professional criteria

These criteria recognise that courses, such as medicine, must reflect explicit legal and professional requirements before practice is permitted:

- Content must provide the kinds of theoretical and practical experiences required for registration.
- Content should include attention to professional ethics.

Psychological criteria

These criteria relate to the application of psychological principles – especially of learning theory – to teaching:

- Content should be carefully integrated to avoid fragmentation and consequential loss of opportunities for students to develop 'deep' approaches to learning (see Chapter 1).
- Content selection must provide opportunities to emphasise and to develop higher-level intellectual skills such as reasoning, problem-solving, critical thinking and creativity.
- Content should provide opportunities for the development of attitudes and values.
- Content should be selected to assist in the development of students as independent lifelong learners.

Practical criteria

These criteria concern the feasibility of teaching something and may relate to resource considerations:

- Content may be derived from one or two major texts because of a lack of suitable alternative materials.
- Content should be influenced by the availability of teaching resources: library materials, information-technology resources, people, patients, physical environment, etc.

Student criteria

These criteria relate to the characteristics of the students you teach. We consider these criteria to be so important that a full section is devoted to them. Student criteria may affect the choice of content (and ways of teaching and assessing) in a variety of ways:

- Content may be selected to reflect the background, needs and interests of all students.
- Content should be matched to the intellectual and maturity level of students.
- Content might take account of the diverse life experiences of students.

How you actually go about selecting content will largely be determined by the kind of person you are (especially by your views about the relative importance of your role as a teacher, the role of students and course content), and the norms and practices in the discipline you teach.

STUDENTS

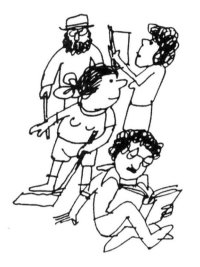

Taking account of student characteristics, needs, and interests is the most difficult part of course planning. The reason for this is that teachers now face increasingly heterogeneous groups of students and, at the same time, must take account of legislative requirements to address specific issues such as occupational health and equal opportunities. It is no longer enough to state that planners need to 'take account of students' and then to proceed as if they did not exist. Experience shows that students can provide invaluable assistance in course planning by consulting them formally and informally.

'Taking account' of students is partly your responsibility and partly your institution's responsibility. Institutional responsibilities – which we would encourage you to influence positively – might include:

★ tutorial assistance in the English language, especially for non-native speakers and international students;
★ bridging courses and foundation courses to assist in the process of adjustment to higher education.

Your responsibilities are no less onerous. In addition to accommodating the wide range of personalities, learning styles, social backgrounds, expectations and academic achievement of normal or direct-entry students from school you must also be prepared to teach students from other backgrounds and with 'different' characteristics than your own. Five examples of current concern which we will briefly discuss are: women, mature-age students, students with a disability, first-year students and international students.

Women students

The role of women and women students in higher education has received a lot of attention. In medical schools in many countries woman are forming an increasingly high proportion of student intakes. However, as the proportion of women in senior clinical and academic positions remains a minority the propensity for bias remains. In course planning you should ensure:

★ the elimination of sexist language in course materials and in teaching.
★ compliance with institutional policies in relation to equal opportunities.

Adult (mature-age) students

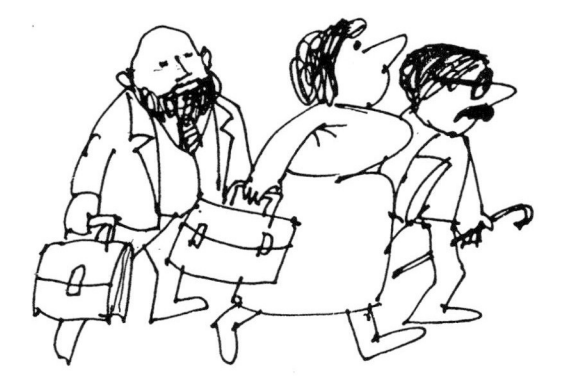

Most medical schools aim to recruit a proportion of mature age students, often from diverse backgrounds. There is also a growing trend towards graduate entry medical schools (outside North America where this has been the norm for many years).

This group brings a rich diversity of experiences and issues. Older students usually approach higher education with a greater intensity of purpose than their younger peers because so much more, in terms of sacrifices and ambitions, rests on their study and achievements. They also expect staff to be more flexible and adaptive in their teaching and assessment methods. These students often experience greater anxiety over assessment arrangements. Vagueness on your part, or in the course plan, can only contribute to this concern.

Students with a disability

You will encounter students with physical impairments, who have medical, psychiatric or psychological problems, or who have a learning disability. Most universities have policies and support arrangements relating to students who have disabilities of these kinds, and we urge you to understand the resources that are available to help you when teaching and assessing such students.

First-year students

The teaching of this group is of particular concern because of their need to adjust to the learning environment of higher education. Some students will belong to a group with specific needs (e.g. mature-age or international students). The sensitive use of small group work (see Chapter 3) can be a means of dealing with some matters, but not all. The selection of content – taking care to induct students into the language and peculiarities of the subject and to the assessment methods – and above all, the clarity of your expectations can all contribute to a smooth and successful transition.

International students

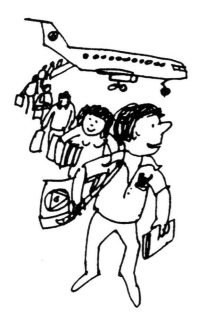

International students, especially those in their first year of studies, require special consideration. These considerations relate most closely to matters of your personal preparation for teaching. Two important aspects are your own level of cultural awareness and the way in which you teach. Cultural awareness can be developed through training programmes, but a more realistic approach for the busy teacher is to develop out-of-class contact with relevant overseas student groups and through reading. The usual principles of good teaching apply as much for this group as for others but particular care should be given to your use of language – especially your speed, pronunciation and use of unnecessarily complex sentence constructions.

As you review these considerations for each group of students you will realise that almost all are worthwhile principles for planning and teaching *all* students and should therefore be taken into account in routine course planning.

In summary, we offer the following general suggestion: be aware of your own attitudes and behaviour, be available and helpful to *all* students and, particularly be willing to learn, to adapt and to adjust. A tall order, we know. But elsewhere in this book you will find suggestions on ways of developing these qualities. Of particular relevance is Chapter 1 on student learning.

As we remarked in our introduction, there is no straightforward formula to guide you in curriculum and course planning. Nowhere is this more evident than in the process of linking the many content and student considerations we have been discussing to the particulars of preparing a course plan. We suggest that you generate a simple checklist of content and student matters to be taken into account during the next step of planning – writing course objectives.

AIMS AND OBJECTIVES

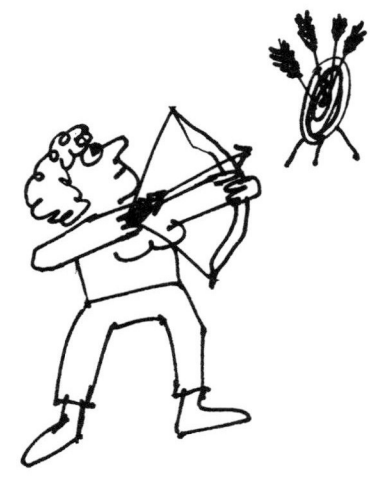

The intentions of the course are usually expressed in the form of aims and objectives. Aims are general statements of intent. Objectives are rather more specific statements of what students should be able to do as a result of a course of study. We are convinced that clear *outcome* objectives are a fundamental tool in course planning because they enable the rational choice of content and teaching and learning activities and are important in planning a valid assessment. Objectives provide a guide to teachers and to students, but should not be so restrictive as to prevent the spontaneity that is so essential to the higher education of students. The relationship between objectives, teaching and learning activities, and assessment is best set out in a course-planning chart such as that seen in Figure 6.1.

Each defined objective is matched with appropriate teaching and learning activities and with a valid form of assessment. For instance, in the example, you would not expect the students to learn to be able to 'take a comprehensive history at the completion of the course' on the basis of lectures, nor would you expect that this could be validly assessed by a paper-and-pencil test. The course designer has provided a relevant teaching and learning activity and a suitable form of assessment.

WRITING OBJECTIVES

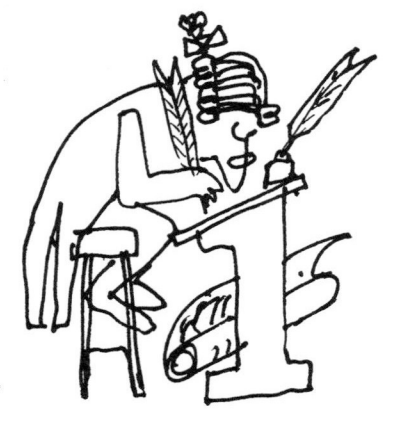

Before you start writing objectives it might help to know what they look like. Here are some examples:

★ Know the basic terminology of the subject
★ Understand the environmental factors which predispose people to lung cancer

★ Obtain a problem-orientated history from a patient
★ Perform a venepuncture
★ Demonstrate a willingness to be critically evaluated by peers.

FIGURE 6.1.
EXAMPLE OF A COURSE PLANNING CHART

OBJECTIVES	TEACHING AND LEARNING ACTIVITIES	ASSESSMENTS
AT THE COMPLETION OF THE COURSE THE STUDENT WILL BE ABLE TO:		
1 TAKE A COMPREHENSIVE HISTORY	**1** PRECEPTOR SESSIONS WITH REVIEW OF VIDEO RECORDINGS OF PATIENT INTERVIEWS	**1** PRECEPTOR'S JUDGEMENT BASED ON VIDEO RECORDINGS OF A HISTORY AT THE END OF THE COURSE
2 **3**	**2** **3**	**2** **3**

In each case, the objective contains a statement which suggests the kind of behaviour that students will be required to demonstrate in order to show that the objective has been achieved. Now, if you look at each objective again, you will notice that they suggest rather different kinds of behaviour. The first two objectives require information of an intellectual kind for their achievement and may be classified as **knowledge objectives**. The third and fourth objectives refer to skills of a practical kind and are thus described as a **skill objectives**. The fifth objective suggests an attitude of mind and is therefore classified as an **attitudinal objective**.

The three broad divisions – knowledge, skills and attitudes – are often used in grouping objectives but you may come across several refinements of each division in the literature. The most common of these refinements is the taxonomy developed by Bloom and his colleagues. They call the three divisions 'domains': cognitive (knowledge and intellectual skills), psychomotor (physical skills) and affective (feelings and attitudes). These domains have been further subdivided to provide hierarchies of objectives of increasing complexity.

Knowledge objectives (the cognitive domain): it is in this area that Bloom's taxonomy has been most widely applied. He proposes six levels:

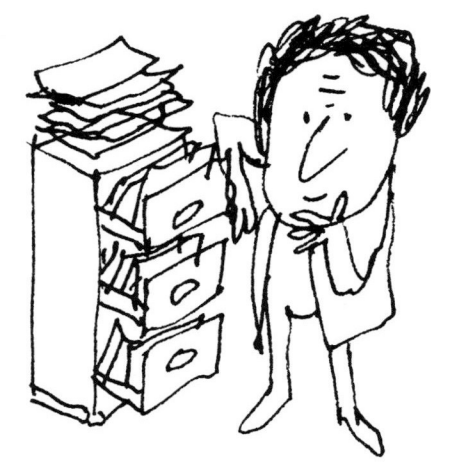

- knowledge;
- comprehension;
- application;
- analysis;
- synthesis; and
- evaluation.

The reason for keeping different levels in mind when writing objectives is that courses sometimes pay undue attention to one level (usually the recall of information).

Skill objectives (the psychomotor domain): in many medical courses, teachers need to pay a great deal of attention to developing skill objectives. Such objectives may be improved if the condition under which the performance is to occur, and the criteria of acceptable performance, can be indicated. You might find it useful to specify the expected level of competent performance. For example there will be some skills with which one would expect students to show a high degree of competence and others with which one might only expect familiarity.

Attitudinal objectives (the affective domain): writing objectives in the affective area is very difficult, which possibly explains whey they are so often ignored. This is unfortunate because, implicity or explicitly, there are many attitudinal qualities we hope to see in our graduating students.

One way of doing so is to attempt to define the starting attitudes of the students and match these with more desirable attitudes towards which you would hope they would move. For example, you might start by assuming that the students had a stereotyped attitude. You would then wish to move them away from this towards an attitude which demonstrated understanding and acceptance of other views. The advantage of this method is that it recognises that not all students will develop the desired attitude nor will they all necessarily start a course with the same attitudes. The way to express objectives using this approach is to state 'Away from . . . (a particular attitude), towards . . . (a desirable attitude)'.

Where do objectives come from?

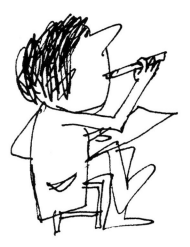

Writing objectives is not simply a process of sitting, pen in hand, waiting for inspiration, although original thinking is certainly encouraged. Objectives will come from a careful consideration of the subject matter, what you and your colleagues know about the students, and about the subject. This will not be an easy task. You should consider a wide range of sources for objectives. These include:

- an analysis of your own and colleagues' knowledge, skills and attitudes;
- ways of thinking and problem-solving to be developed;
- students' interests, needs and characteristics;
- subject matter, as reflected in the published literature (especially in suitable textbooks);
- the needs of patients and the community;
- the requirements of professional certifying authorities;
- the objectives of the department or school.

How specific and detailed should objectives be?

This is a question frequently asked. The answer depends on the purposes for which the objectives are to be used. In designing a course, the objectives will be more general than the objectives for a particular teaching session within the course. As objective writing can become tedious, trivial and time-consuming it is best to keep your objectives simple, unambiguous and broad enough to convey clearly your intentions. To illustrate from our own field of teaching, the objectives for a six-week clinical skills course, conducted for groups of 9-10 students, are shown below. Though quite broad, these objectives have proved detailed enough for course planning purposes and for making the intentions of the programme clear to students.

FIGURE 6.2.
EXAMPLE OF COURSE OBJECTIVES

OBJECTIVES	TEACHING AND LEARNING ACTIVITIES	ASSESSMENTS
AT THE COMPLETION OF THE COURSE THE STUDENT WILL WILL BE BE ABLE TO:		
1 TAKE A COMPREHENSIVE HISTORY	**1**	**1**
2 PERFORM A COMPLETE PHYSICAL EXAMINATION	**2**	**2**
3 WRITE UP THE HISTORY AND EXAMINATION AND CONSTRUCT A PROBLEM LIST	**3**	**3**
4 MAKE DECISIONS ON DIAGNOSIS, INVESTIGATIONS AND MANAGEMENT	**4**	**4**
5 RELATE WELL TO PATIENTS	**5**	**5**
6 SHOW THAT HE/SHE HAS IMPROVED HIS/HER KNOWLEDGE OF MEDICINE AND SURGERY	**6**	**6**

CHOOSING METHODS AND RELATING OBJECTIVES TO TEACHING AND LEARNING ACTIVITIES

The methods you employ to achieve the objectives should not only allow those objectives to be realised, but will also reflect the kind of orientation you have to course planning. If your orientation is primarily the transmission of content, it is likely that your teaching methods will be dominated by lectures, assigned reading of books and electronically based materials, and set problem-solving exercises. If it is to be the intellectual and personal development of your students, small group teaching or individual tutorials and e-mail discussions are likely to play a more important role.

The actual choice of methods will be governed by several factors. Among the most important will be:

- ensuring that students engage in appropriate learning activities;
- your own expertise in using different methods;
- technical and financial resources to support the method you wish to use.

Before leaving this subject we should like you to consider one important matter about choice of methods. Courses are often constructed in ways that reveal a growing complexity of subject matter. For example, early in the first year there may be an emphasis on basic principles and ideas. In later years, subject matter may be very much more complex and demanding. Yet, in our experience, the teaching methods often used in the later years do not generally demand higher levels of intellectual performance and personal involvement.

The main types of teaching in medical education, such as lecturing, small group teaching and clinical teaching are dealt with in earlier chapters. These are by no means all of the methods available. Other possibilities include project work, peer teaching and a variety of technology-based techniques. In addition, it should be remembered that students undertake many learning activities in the absence of teaching and there is growing pressure for this to become more common. It is reasonable to make explicit in your objectives areas where you expect the students to work on their own. This particularly applies to knowledge objectives which might be achieved just as well independently in the library or by accessing the Web. It could also apply to some skill objectives where students might be expected to seek out relevant experience by themselves or in open access skills laboratories.

The way in which this process has been followed through in the clinical skills course we have already introduced is demonstrated once again on the course planning chart (Figure 6.3). When planning this course we were aware that many students needed assistance with their basic

FIGURE 6.3.
EXAMPLE OF MATCHING TEACHING AND LEARNING ACTIVITIES TO COURSE OBJECTIVES

OBJECTIVES	TEACHING AND LEARNING ACTIVITIES	ASSESSMENTS
AT THE COMPLETION OF THE COURSE THE STUDENT WILL BE ABLE TO:		
1 TAKE A COMPREHENSIVE HISTORY	**1** PRECEPTOR SESSIONS WITH REVIEW OF VIDEO RECORDINGS OF PATIENT INTERVIEWS	
2 PERFORM A COMPLETE PHYSICAL EXAMINATION	**2** VIEWING DEMONSTRATION VIDEOTAPE. PRECEPTOR SESSIONS WITH PATIENTS. WARD PRACTICE. WARD ROUNDS WITH RESIDENT STAFF	
3 WRITE UP THE HISTORY AND EXAMINATION AND CONSTRUCT A PROBLEM LIST	**3** HAND-OUT OF EXEMPLAR CASE HISTORY WRITE-UPS ON WARD PATIENTS PRECEPTOR SESSIONS TO CHECK AND DISCUSS WRITE-UPS	
4 MAKE DECISIONS ON DIAGNOSIS, INVESTIGATIONS AND MANAGEMENT	**4** PROBLEM-BASED WHOLE GROUP DISCUSSION SESSIONS REVIEW OF CASE WRITE-UPS	
5 RELATE WELL TO PATIENTS	**5** PRECEPTOR SESSIONS WITH REVIEW OF VIDEO RECORDINGS OF PATIENT INTERVIEWS	
6 SHOW THAT HE/SHE HAS IMPROVED HIS/HER KNOWLEDGE OF MEDICINE AND SURGERY	**6** INDEPENDENT LEARNING. PREPARATION OF CASES FOR PRESENTATION. COMPUTERIZED SELF-ASSESSMENT PROGRAMMES	

history-taking and physical examination skills. We thus decided to put the majority of our staff time into achieving the first two objectives. The most appropriate teaching method was obviously direct observation with feedback and as this is very time-consuming we opted for a preceptor system where one staff member was responsible for only three students throughout the programme. However, opportunity was also provided for students to obtain additional ward practice on their own and with the resident staff. Senior students were also mobilised to provide further help and instruction in this area. One of the implications of this decision on staff allocation was to accept that the sixth objective (improving their knowledge in the subjects Medicine and Surgery) would have to be achieved by other methods. This has involved an expectation that students accept responsibility for doing much of this themselves. We have also designed and prepared a variety of self-instructional materials. Other teaching techniques are incorporated to achieve other objectives.

RELATING OBJECTIVES TO ASSESSMENT METHODS

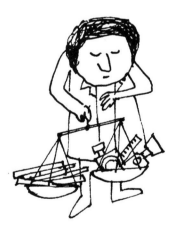

While it is obviously important to match the teaching and learning activities with the objectives, it is absolutely vital to match the assessment methods to the objectives and to the teaching and learning activities. Failure to do so is the reason why many courses fail to live up to expectations. A mismatch of assessment and objectives may lead to serious distortions of student learning because, whether we like it or not, what is present in the assessments will drive what most students set out to learn.

In designing your course, we believe that it is also important to distinguish carefully between two types of assessment. One is primarily designed to give feedback to the students as they go along (**formative assessment**). The other is to assess their abilities for the purposes of decision making or grading (**summative assessment**). Formative assessment is a crucial part of the educational process, especially where complex intellectual and practical skills are to be mastered. Such assessment is notoriously deficient in medical schools, particularly in regard to clinical teaching (see Chapter 5).

The way in which assessment was designed in the example of our clinical skills course is shown in Figure 6.4. As no formal examination is required at the completion of the course, the major emphasis of the assessment activities is formative. However, assessment activities of a summative type are conducted during the final two weeks of the programme when aspects of the students' performance are observed by preceptors and by other staff members. You will note that the assessment of knowledge is left largely to the students themselves. In other circumstances we might have used a written test to assess this component of the course.

SEQUENCING AND ORGANISING THE COURSE

It is unlikely that the way in which you have set out your objectives, teaching and assessment on the planning chart will be the best chronological or practical way to present the course to students. There are several other things that must be done. First, there must be a **grouping** of related objectives and activities. (In the example we are following throughout this chapter, such a grouping occurs for objectives one to the three which are largely to be achieved by the preceptor sessions.) Secondly, there must be **sequencing** of the teaching activities. There are likely to be circumstances in your own context that influence you to sequence a course in a particular way, such as semesters or teaching terms. However, there are also a number of educational grounds upon which to base the sequencing. These include:

- Proceeding from what students know to what they do not know;
- Proceeding from concrete experiences to abstract reasoning;
- The logical or historical development of a subject;
- Prioritising important themes or concepts;
- Starting from unusual, novel or complex situations and working backwards towards understanding (e.g. as in problem-based learning).

As our understanding of how different factors can influence learning advances, you should give consideration to the ways in which you can facilitate deep-learning approaches by your students through the way in which you organise

FIGURE 6.4.
EXAMPLES OF MATCHING ASSESSMENT PROCEDURES TO COURSE OBJECTIVES

OBJECTIVES	TEACHING AND LEARNING ACTIVITIES	ASSESSMENTS
AT THE COMPLETION OF THE COURSE THE STUDENT WILL BE ABLE TO:		
1 TAKE A COMPREHENSIVE HISTORY	1 PRECEPTOR SESSIONS WITH REVIEW OF VIDEO RECORDING OF PATIENT INTERVIEWS.	1 ASSESSMENT OF VIDEO RECORDING DURING COURSE (FORMATIVE). ASSESSMENT OF VIDEO RECORDING AT END OF COURSE (SUMMATIVE)
2 PERFORM A COMPLETE PHYSICAL EXAMINATION.	2 VIEWING DEMONSTRATION VIDEO TAPE. PRECEPTOR SESSIONS WITH PATIENTS WARD PRACTICE WARD ROUNDS WITH RESIDENT STAFF	2 DIRECT OBSERVATION DURING COURSE (FORMATIVE). DIRECT OBSERVATION AT END OF THE COURSE (SUMMATIVE)
3 WRITE UP THE HISTORY AND EXAMINATION AND CONSTRUCT A PROBLEM LIST	3 HANDOUT OF EXEMPLAR CASE HISTORY WRITE-UPS ON WARD PATIENTS. PRECEPTOR SESSIONS TO CHECK AND DISCUSS WRITE-UPS	3 MARKING AND DISCUSSION OF CASE WRITE-UPS (FORMATIVE). MARKING OF CASE WRITE-UPS AT END OF COURSE (SUMMATIVE)
4 MAKE DECISIONS ON DIAGNOSIS, INVESTIGATIONS AND MANAGEMENT	4 PROBLEM-BASED WHOLE GROUP DISCUSSION SESSIONS. REVIEW OF CASE WRITE-UPS	4 PERFORMANCE IN WHOLE GROUP SESSIONS (SUMMATIVE)
5 RELATE WELL TO PATIENTS	5 PRECEPTOR SESSIONS WITH REVIEW OF VIDEO-RECORDINGS OF PATIENT INTERVIEWS	5 ASSESSMENT OF VIDEO RECORDING DURING COURSE (FORMATIVE AND SUMMATIVE)
6 SHOW THAT HE/SHE HAS IMPROVED HIS/HER KNOWLEDGE OF MEDICINE AND SURGERY	6 INDEPENDENT LEARNING. PREPARATION OF CASES FOR PRESENTATION	6 SELF-ASSESSMENT. COMPUTERIZED SELF-ASSESSMENT PROGRAMMES (FORMATIVE)

and manage the course and the kinds of intellectual and assessment demands you place on them. We suggest that you review the relevant sections in Chapter 1 to guide you in this matter.

Finally, you will need to consider the broad organising principles behind your course. Will you, for example, offer it in a traditional way with a set timetable of carefully sequenced learning activities culminating in an end-of-year examination? Or will you design your course more flexibly around a completely different approach such as problem-based learning?

OTHER COURSE DESIGN CONSIDERATIONS

Many of the important educational considerations in designing a course have been addressed, but there are other matters that must be dealt with before a course can be mounted. These are only briefly described because the way in which they are handled depends very much on the administrative arrangements of the particular situation in which you teach. Having said that, we are not suggesting in any way that your educational plans must be subservient to administrative considerations. Clearly, in the best of all possible worlds, the administrative considerations would be entirely subservient to the educational plans but the reality is that there will be a series of trade-offs, with educational considerations hopefully paramount.

In planning your new course, you will need to take the following into account.

Administrative responsibilities: it will be necessary for one person to assume the responsibility of course co-ordination. This job will require the scheduling of teachers, students, teaching activities, assessment time and re-sources.

Allocation of time: many courses are over ambitious and require far more time (often on the part of the students) for their completion than is reasonable. This is especially true of parts of a larger course of study. In allocating time, you will need to consider the total time available and its breakdown, and how time is to be spent in the course. It is often desirable to use blocks of time to deal with a particular topic, rather than 'spinning it out' over a term, semester or year.

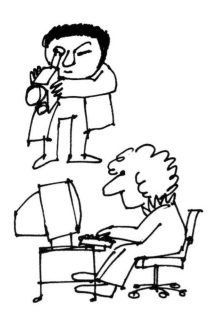

Allocation of teaching rooms, clinics, laboratories and equipment: courses depend for their success on the careful allocation of resources. It is important that all competing claims are settled early so that orderly teaching can take place.

Technical and administrative support: whether you teach a course alone, or as one of a team, you will find a need for support of some kind or other. It may be as simple as the services of someone to prepare course notes and examination papers, or as complex as requiring, at different times, the assistance of technicians and laboratory staff. Your needs for support must be considered at the planning stage.

EVALUATING THE COURSE

Many teachers may find a discussion of course evaluation in a chapter on planning rather odd, perhaps believing that this activity is something that takes place after a course has been completed. We believe that this generally should not be the case. It is our contention that in teaching you should continually evaluate what you are doing and how the course design and plans are working out in practice. In this way, modification and adjustments can be made in a systematic and informed manner. But what is evaluation? You will often find the terms 'evaluation' and 'assessment' used interchangeably, but evaluation is generally understood to refer to the process of obtaining information about a course (or teaching) for subsequent judgement and decision-making. This process, properly done, will involve you in rather more than handing around a student questionnaire during the last lecture. What you do clearly depends on what you want to find out, but thorough course planning and course revision will require information about three different aspects of your course. These are the context of and inputs into your course; the processes of teaching, learning, assessment and course administration; and, finally, the outcomes of the course.

Context and input evaluation: this is crucial if mistakes and problems are not to be attributed, unfairly, to teachers. In this type of evaluation you will need to consider the course in relation to such matters as other related courses, the entering abilities and characteristics of students, the resources and equipment available to teach with, and the overall design and planning arrangement for the course. The major sources of information you can use here will be in the form of course documents, student records, financial statements and the like.

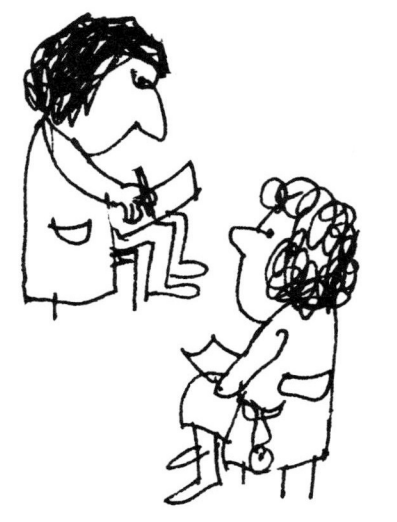

Process evaluation: this focuses on the conduct of the teaching, learning, assessment and administration. It is here that the views of students can be sought as they are the only people who experience the full impact of teaching in the course. Questionnaires, written statements, interviews and discussion are techniques that you can consider.

Outcome evaluation: this looks at student attainments at the end of the course. Naturally you will review the results of assessment and judge whether they meet with the implied and expressed hopes for the course. Discussion with students and observation of aspects of their behaviour will help you determine their attitudes to the course you taught.

In all evaluations, whether of a course or of teaching, it is helpful to keep in mind that there are many sources of information available to you and a variety of methods you can use. We suggest that you look at Chapter 10 on evaluation for more information about this.

GUIDED READING

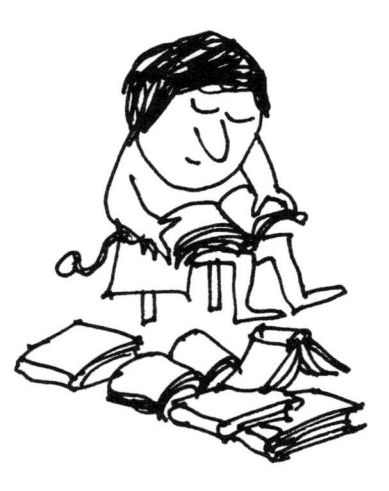

For a useful extension of the material in this chapter we suggest you have a look at S. Toohey's *Designing Courses for Higher Education*, SRHE and Open University Press, Buckingham, 1999 and J. Biggs' *Teaching for Quality Learning at University: What the Student Does*, SRHE and Open University Press, Buckingham, 1999.

For a clear and systematic guide to curriculum planning we recommend *Planning a Professional Curriculum* by L. Fisher and C. Levene, University of Calgary Press, 1989. If you wish more detailed guidance on objectives we suggest N. Gronlund, *How to Write Instructional Objectives*, Prentice Hall Inc, Englewood Cliffs, 1995.

Books and articles referred to in this chapter

B. Bloom et al. *Taxonomy of Educational Objectives*. Handbook I: Cognitive Domain. McKay, New York, 1956.

7:   TEACHING IN A PROBLEM-BASED COURSE

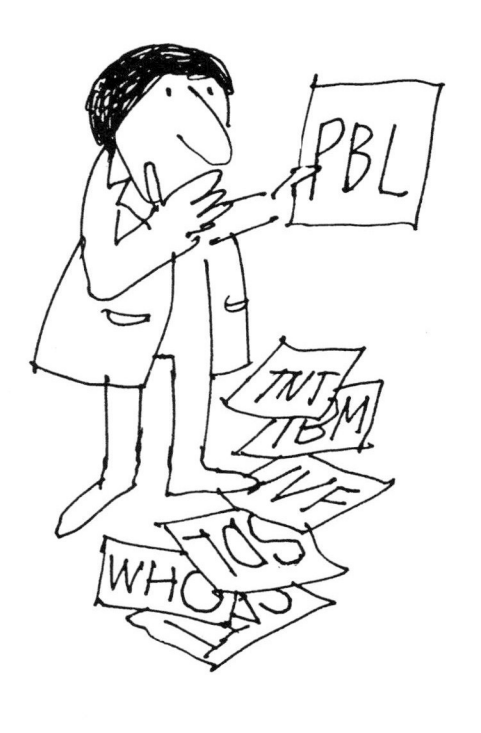

INTRODUCTION

Until recently the vast majority of medical teachers were working in traditional medical schools and unlikely to be challenged by alternative teaching methods which were to be found only in a small minority of radical, and usually new, medical schools. However, a dramatic change has occurred. Many conventional and well-established medical schools have undertaken curriculum reviews and have decided to change to 'problem-based learning' (PBL). However, experience has shown that when this approach has been introduced its effectiveness has often been undermined by a lack of understanding of the purpose and process of PBL. This chapter aims to give you guidance if faced with teaching in a problem-based course. It will not attempt to debate the rationale behind PBL in any depth nor will it analyse the research on its effectiveness. The Guided Reading will provide a starting point if you wish to pursue these issues.

WHAT IS PROBLEM-BASED LEARNING?

The traditional way of medical school teaching has been to require students to undertake sequential courses in the pre-clinical and para-clinical sciences as a prerequisite to commencing studies in the medical sciences and clinical practice. Such courses have been the autonomous responsibility of academic departments who have jealously guarded their curriculum time and their control over course content and examinations. The degree of integration, particularly in the pre-clinical disciplines, has often been limited. This structure has formed the basis of the curriculum for most medical schools since the Flexner report in 1910 but is starting to collapse in the face of the intolerable load of information that each discipline expects the student to learn. The veritable explosion of scientific knowledge relevant to medicine, and the increasing specialisation of clinical practice, has led to unmanageable requests for the inclusion of more courses and more content without agreement or action on what is to be excluded. Efforts to deal with these issues using strategies such as organ systems teaching have made little impact. An alternative approach has become necessary and PBL is one gaining increasing acceptance.

In brief, the approach is one in which learning is based around problems, usually written clinical cases. Students work through these problems, under greater or lesser degree of guidance from tutors, defining what they do not know and what they need to know in order to understand (not necessarily just to solve) the problem. The justification for this is firmly based in modern psychological theories of learning which have determined that knowledge is remembered and recalled more effectively if learning is based in the context in which it is going to be used in the future. Thus, if basic science knowledge is structured around representations of cases likely to be encountered in medical practice in the future, it is more likely to be remembered. Problem-based learning is also inherently integrative with the need to understand relevant aspects of anatomy, physiology, biochemistry, pathology and so on being readily apparent in each case.

There is some evidence that students do, in the long term, recall more information in the context of patient problems when taught in the PBL way when compared with students taught in the disciplinary-based way. What is strikingly apparent is that students prefer this approach and become much more motivated to learn, a prerequisite to the desirable deep approach to learning discussed in Chapter 1. Other educational objectives believed to be addressed by PBL are, according to Barrows, the development of effective clinical reasoning skills and self directed learning skills. However, several recent reviews in the literature reveal little evidence of major differences between graduates from schools with a problem-based curriculum and those from schools with a more traditional curriculum. Whether this is actually true or reflects limitations of the indicators used to evaluate outcomes is unclear. Whatever trends there are generally seem to favour PBL.

IMPLEMENTATING PROBLEM-BASED LEARNING

Problem-based learning will have different implications if you are involved on a curriculum committee than if your involvement is as a tutor to a group of students undertaking a PBL exercise. In the former situation you will be engaged in reviewing the evidence for the effectiveness of PBL, in discussing the politics and practicalities of making such a major change to the curriculum, and in conducting or arranging information sessions and workshops for the staff of the medical school in order to gain their support.

Having decided in principle to proceed, your school may choose one of several implementation models (Figure 7.1).

FIGURE 7.1.
MODELS FOR CHANGE TO
PROBLEM-BASED LEARNING

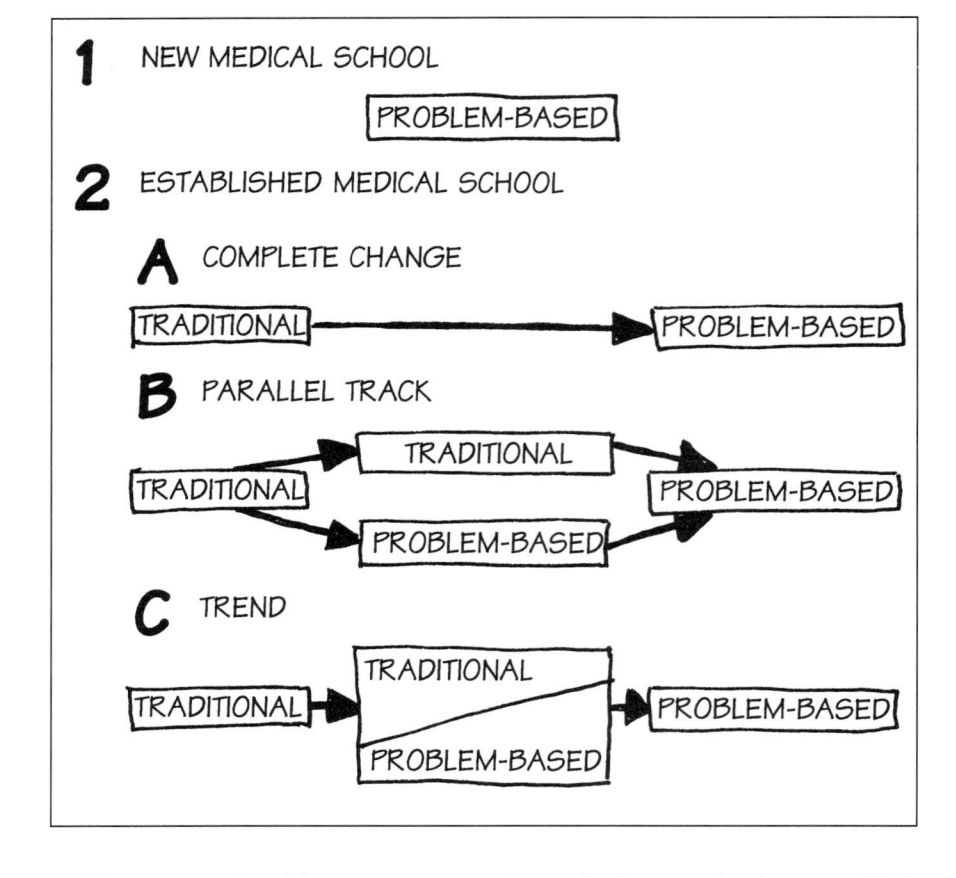

You may decide to convert the whole curriculum to PBL along the lines of the innovative schools of which McMaster University in Canada is the exemplar. Alternatively you may want to follow the path of schools such as New Mexico or Harvard and commence with two tracks, running the PBL track parallel to the conventional track with the advantage of gaining experience and undertaking comparative evaluation. If you wish to be more cautious another alternative is to introduce PBL as a component of the curriculum or into individual courses with or without the expectation that the whole course will eventually change to PBL.

COURSE DESIGN CONSIDERATIONS

The basic principles of course design are the same as those in any other course (see Chapter 6). There is no single best way of approaching this task and it will be important to

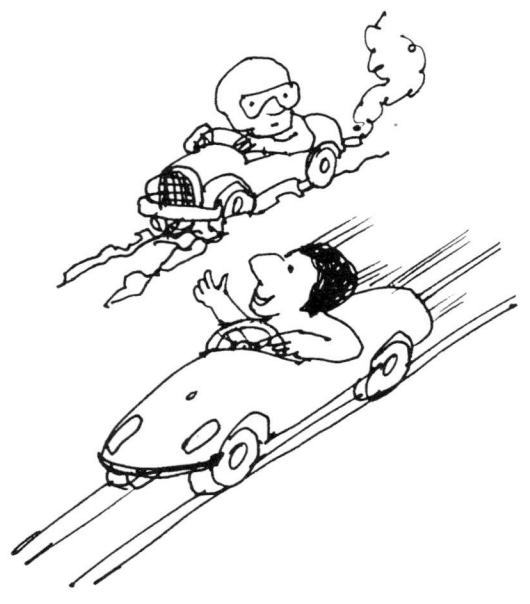

ascertain which of the many styles of PBL you are expected to implement. In general, PBL curricula are constructed in a modular format with blocks of several weeks being committed to a common theme (e.g. gastroenterological problems; reproduction). Factors to be taken into account will include:

The major purposes of the module

There are generally two major purposes to be achieved in a PBL module. One is the attainment of specific learning objectives in the form of an integrated knowledge and understanding of a defined problem (e.g. diarrhoea). The other is skill in the process of problem-solving and self-directed learning.

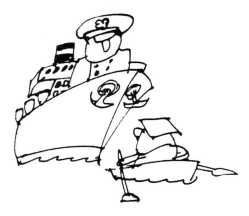

These are combined in various proportions in the **Guided Discovery** and **Open Discovery** approaches. In the Guided Discovery approach the emphasis is on both content and process. The course is carefully structured as a series of modules containing problems which direct students into learning the appropriate basic science and clinical content. While it is essential to allow the students to discover the learning issues from the problem, written guidelines are provided and tutor prompting occurs to ensure that all content areas are considered.

The Open Discovery approach places more emphasis on the process. The framework of the course and the problems may be the same as in the Guided Discovery approach but the students have much greater responsibility for determining what they should learn. Complete coverage of all content aspects is not expected.

The method of instruction

PBL is usually conducted in small groups consisting of 5-10 students with a tutor. As a rule, the tutor is there to facilitate the process rather than to be a provider of content knowledge. In some schools tutors are deliberately chosen to be non-experts particularly where the Open Discovery approach is predominant. Small group activities are supported by independent study for which curriculum time must be carefully protected. Where tutor resources are limited it is possible to conduct PBL in large group settings using student-led groups for discussion or by relying to a greater degree on independent study. We have used this approach successfully in a foundation course using PBL for first-year medical students (see later).

The selection of the problems

This is one of the most important considerations in course design. The problems must be of the kind that will ultimately be faced by the students after they graduate but must also be both broad enough and specific enough to engage the students in learning activities which match the curriculum objectives. They should not be answerable by simple responses. In general they should be patient problems or health problems which will require students to go through the following process:

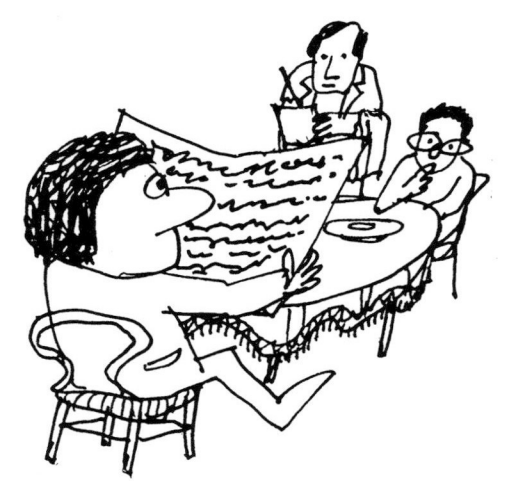

- Analysis of the problem.
- Identification of the multidisciplinary knowledge required to understand and solve the problem.
- Obtaining agreement on the independent learning tasks to be performed.
- Obtaining agreement on when the learning tasks will be achieved.
- Application of the newly acquired knowledge to the initial problem.
- Further cycles of the process if necessary.

While these problems will usually be represented in written form every chance should be taken to engage the students in the same PBL process with real problems encountered in the health care setting. To this end clinical teachers should be actively engaged in supporting the programme. This can be particularly helpful in the earlier parts of the curriculum where opportunities for clinical experience may be more limited. Increasingly, the computer is being used to manage and support PBL.

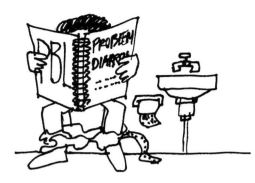

Preparing the PBL modules

You may be asked to prepare one or more of these modules. Your first task will be to obtain the objectives if they have been prepared by an overseeing group. More likely you will have to develop them yourself. Such objectives should define what it is the students should have achieved when they have completed the module (see Chapter 6). It is important to seek the involvement of teachers from all the disciplines that are expected to contribute to the learning outcome of the students.

Once objectives are agreed, case summaries must be carefully prepared, remembering that they should be interesting and complex enough to engage students in the problem-solving process. A written guide should be developed for the tutors involved in the module, its content depending to some extent on the familiarity they are likely to have with the problem. An abbreviated example of such a guide is illustrated in Figure 7.2.

Resource materials for students and tutors should be identified (e.g. references, weblinks, audio-visual materials, computer simulations, static demonstrations and even lectures). Resource people who could be available for students to contact should be approached and times that meetings with students could be scheduled should be ascertained. An alternative is to use email or an on-line discussion group.

Assessment

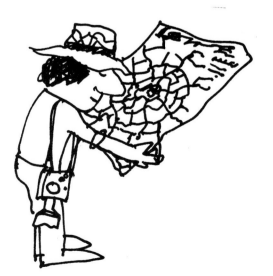

This is one area where there is still considerable debate and development. It is important to involve all disciplines in the preparation of assessment materials as it is to engage them in defining the objectives. Only in this way will they be convinced that their discipline is being adequately represented. This reassurance is particularly important to the basic scientists who are often those most threatened by a change to PBL.

The most important focus for assessment in PBL is formative. Constantly challenging the students to evaluate the success of their learning is a vital role of the tutor.

FIGURE 7.2.
OUTLINE OF TUTOR GUIDE TO
MODULE AIMS

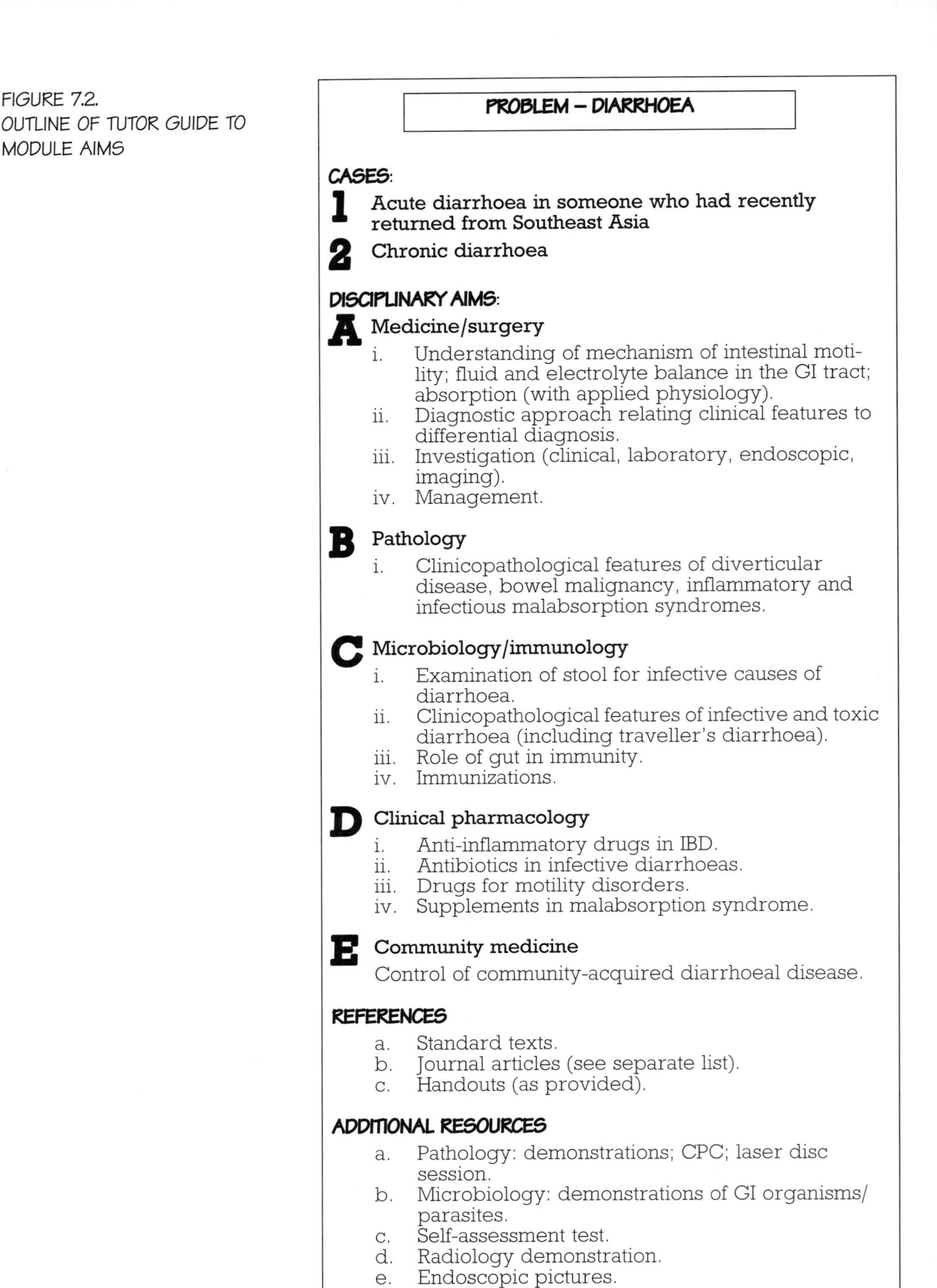

PROBLEM – DIARRHOEA

CASES:

1 Acute diarrhoea in someone who had recently returned from Southeast Asia

2 Chronic diarrhoea

DISCIPLINARY AIMS:

A Medicine/surgery

    i.   Understanding of mechanism of intestinal motility; fluid and electrolyte balance in the GI tract; absorption (with applied physiology).

    ii. Diagnostic approach relating clinical features to differential diagnosis.

    iii. Investigation (clinical, laboratory, endoscopic, imaging).

    iv. Management.

B Pathology

    i.   Clinicopathological features of diverticular disease, bowel malignancy, inflammatory and infectious malabsorption syndromes.

C Microbiology/immunology

    i.   Examination of stool for infective causes of diarrhoea.

    ii. Clinicopathological features of infective and toxic diarrhoea (including traveller's diarrhoea).

    iii. Role of gut in immunity.

    iv. Immunizations.

D Clinical pharmacology

    i.   Anti-inflammatory drugs in IBD.

    ii. Antibiotics in infective diarrhoeas.

    iii. Drugs for motility disorders.

    iv. Supplements in malabsorption syndrome.

E Community medicine

Control of community-acquired diarrhoeal disease.

REFERENCES

    a. Standard texts.

    b. Journal articles (see separate list).

    c. Handouts (as provided).

ADDITIONAL RESOURCES

    a. Pathology: demonstrations; CPC; laser disc session.

    b. Microbiology: demonstrations of GI organisms/parasites.

    c. Self-assessment test.

    d. Radiology demonstration.

    e. Endoscopic pictures.

Students must also be challenged to develop self-assessment skills. A way of approaching this is outlined in Chapter 8 in the section on self-assessment.

Most schools will also wish to have summative assessment procedures. It cannot be stated too strongly the potential danger this poses. Conventional knowledge-based tests, such as MCQs, should be avoided except perhaps for student self-assessment or progress testing. Unfortunately, test methods more suitable for PBL courses are not well developed. The Modified Essay Question may be the simplest and most flexible format if a written test of integrated knowledge is required (see Chapter 8). In many schools the tutor is asked to rate students on their performance with the emphasis being as much on their group and personal learning skills as on their grasp of the content.

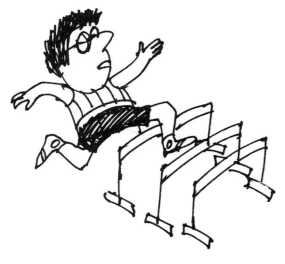

Few methods have been specifically designed to evaluate problem-based self-directed learning skills. The most well known of these is the Triple Jump Test developed at McMaster University. As the name implies this is a three step procedure. In the first step the student works through a theoretical problem on a one-to-one basis with a tutor. The student is asked to think aloud as the problem is assessed and learning needs determined. The second step consists of a fixed period of time (2-3 hours) during which the student may seek out relevant information. The final step involves a return to the tutor where the new information is used to re-analyse the problem and hopefully come to some conclusions. The tutor evaluates the efficiency and effectiveness of the student's problem-solving and self-directed learning skills. These are compared with the student's self-assessment of his or her performance. This method has obvious merit as a formative evaluation but, as there is little information about its validity and reliability, so its value for summative purposes has yet to be established.

To obtain more information on assessment in PBL courses we suggest you look at the book by Boud and Feletti and the review article by Nendaz and Tekian. You will also find it very helpful to contact PBL schools and see what strategies and methods they are using.

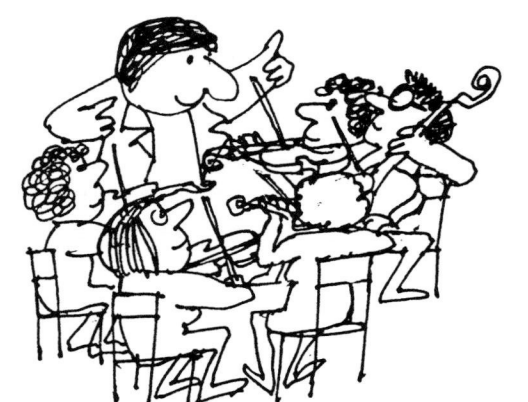

TUTORING

The first task you are likely to have to perform in a PBL course is that of tutor. Your role will generally be one of facilitator rather then expert, a role you may initially find rather difficult. The sessions will usually be conducted in small groups so Chapter 3 may also be helpful.

In brief, your main task is to help your students develop the skills to work effectively as a group member. To do this the student must understand the purpose of their PBL activities and not see the session simply as one of solving the problem. They are usually expected to learn a lot of 'stuff'. The process skills they will need to do this effectively include group skills, information literacy (locating, retrieving, evaluating and using information of all kinds), negotiating, interviewing and presenting. So while you may appear to be teaching your subject less, you should have the pleasure of observing students learn the expected content in a much more interesting and exciting way.

Modules are designed to be completed in a fixed period of time. For the purpose of this chapter the time allocated to a module will be assumed to be one week. A possible model of a week's activities is seen in Figure 7.3.

FIGURE 7.3.
EXAMPLE OF WEEKLY ACTIVITIES IN A PBL COURSE

MONDAY	2.00 – 2.30	INTRODUCTION TO THE 'CASE(S) OF THE WEEK'
	2.30 – 3.15	'CONCEPTS' LECTURE ON MAIN TOPIC(S) OF THE WEEK
	3.45 – 4.30	GROUP MEETINGS (WITH TUTOR) – CLARIFICATION AND ALLOCATION OF CASE-BASED LEARNING TASKS
TUESDAY	2.00 – 5.00	AVAILABILITY OF DEMONSTRATIONS/RESOURCE PEOPLE
WEDNESDAY	2.00	GROUP MEETINGS WITH OR WITHOUT TUTOR – CHECK ON PROGRESS – REFINE LEARNING TASKS
	4.00 – 5.00	CLINICO-PATHOLOGICAL CONFERENCE
THURSDAY	2.00 – 3.00	RECENT ADVANCES LECTURE
FRIDAY	2.00 – 3.30	GROUP MEETINGS (WITH TUTOR) – CHECK ON COMPLETION OF LEARNING TASKS AND PROBLEM SOLUTION – ASSESSMENT OF PROGRESS

FIGURE 7.4.
EXAMPLE OF CASE-BASED
PROBLEM

MR. KIM JONES IS A 46-YEAR-OLD ACCOUNTANT. HE HAD RECENTLY BEEN ON A 6-WEEK TRIP TO SINGAPORE, THAILAND AND NEPAL. WHILE IN THAILAND HE HAD DIARRHOEA FOR TWO DAYS ABOUT THREE DAYS AFTER HIS ARRIVAL. THIS SETTLED DOWN WITHOUT ANY SPECIFIC TREATMENT AND HE CONTINUED ON WITH HIS JOURNEY TO NEPAL SEVERAL DAYS LATER. HE HAD NO FURTHER HEALTH PROBLEMS DURING THE REMAINDER OF THE TRIP.

HE NOW PRESENTS TO HIS DOCTOR TWO MONTHS ATER RETURNING FROM ABROAD. HE IS CONCERNED BECAUSE THE DIARRHOEA RETURNED A MONTH AGO. HE SEEMS ALSO TO BE PASSING A LOT OF WIND AND THE STOOLS HAVE AN OFFENSIVE SMELL. HE IS OTHERWISE QUITE WELL.

At the first session you will introduce the problem. Usually this will be a written case-history (Figure 7.4) but could be supported by a videotape of part of the history or even by a visit to a real patient. One possible way of conducting this session is outlined in Figure 7.5.

FIGURE 7.5.
PROCEDURE FOR
INTRODUCTORY SESSION

Procedure

A Tutor explains that his/her role is primarily as a session facilitator not as an expert on the content.

B Tutor ensures that everyone is introduced if this is a new group.

C Tutor provides students with the module handout which will include the problem case, list of resources, scheduled activities etc.

D Students analyse the problem case, identify learning issues, allocate learning tasks. Tutor ensures all expected outcomes are included.

E Students and tutor agree on future group meeting times.

Students are then engaged in formulating questions about the problem (e.g. What might be the cause of the diarrhoea? Why did it resolve then recur? Why was the stool offensive? What was the mechanism for the diarrhoea? How should it be investigated? etc.). To assist the process you should be provided with additional information about the case (physical examination findings; investigations) to feed into the discussion at the initial session or later in the week. You should also have a list of resources which are relevant to the problem such as books, articles, videotapes, web-based materials and experts available for consultation. There might even be a lecture or two for the students to attend. The expected level of tutor intervention will depend to some extent on whether the approach in your school is Guided or Open Discovery.

When agreement has been reached on the learning tasks to be performed, arrangements are made to meet again during the week to review progress and pool information. You may or may not attend such meetings. Students will determine whether further information is needed and, if so, additional learning tasks will be assigned.

At the end of the week, progress with the problem is reviewed. Remaining difficulties are resolved. At such a time some expertise relating to the problem may be of value. However, complete resolution of the problem is rarely possible nor is it to be seen as the aim. Students should become aware that there is always more to be learned.

If the institution is using expert tutors it is unlikely that you will spend many sessions with one group of students. You may only operate as a tutor for a few weeks a year. On the other hand, if non-expert tutors are the policy then you may be the facilitator to one group for an extended period of time. In many ways this is likely to be more rewarding albeit more time consuming.

STAFF RESOURCES FOR PROBLEM-BASED LEARNING

One of the major concerns for medical schools contemplating changing to PBL is that of staff resources. It is widely perceived that PBL is dependent on small groups and that this will demand more staff or a considerable extra time commitment for existing staff. This may well be true if one is trying to emulate the McMaster model of PBL. However, it is possible for compromises to be made. For instance, if non-expert tutors are acceptable for some components of the course it may be possible to use staff (e.g. laboratory scientists, clinicians) who previously have not had a major teaching role.

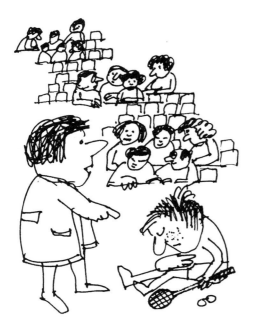

Another alternative is to undertake the normally tutor-led sessions in large group settings. We have some experience of this in a first-year foundation course in which we aim to introduce students to the process of PBL. Clinical problems (e.g. diarrhoea in a traveller; chest pain in a squash player) are introduced to a whole class of students in a lecture theatre session. Students are asked to arrange themselves informally into groups of 4-5. The process of problem analysis is undertaken by these groups, a procedure that produces a rewarding hum of activity in the lecture theatre. The teacher then gathers together the ideas in an interactive manner from representative of the groups. Agreement is reached on the information the students require to proceed with the problem. If the exercise is to be completed in one session this can then be provided by the teacher or an invited colleague who is the 'expert'. On the other hand the full process of PBL can be continued with students departing to report back at a subsequent session having completed their independent learning tasks.

This approach requires skill on the part of the teacher. However, it is one we have found to be very successful and highly rewarding. Student feedback has been very supportive. In a sense it is an extension to the additional techniques referred to in Chapter 2 on Large Group Teaching.

Whatever approach is used the need for effective **staff development** is paramount if PBL is to be successfully implemented. Unfortunately may schools fail in this regard with inevitable disappointment to staff and students. Particularly helpful are workshops in which staff take different roles in a PBL group exercise and observing a real student PBL group in action.

GUIDED READING

There are several books and many articles which provide the necessary background to the philosophy, justification and practice of PBL.

Some of the seminal work in the area was conducted by Barrows and two of his books are recommended. These are H. Barrows and R. Tamblyn, ***Problem-Based Learning:***

An Approach to Medical Education, Springer, New York, 1980 and H. Barrows, *How to Design a Problem-Based Curriculum for Preclinical Years*, Springer, New York, 1985.

A more recent book which provides examples of PBL from many other professions is **The Challenge of Problem-Based Learning** by D. Boud and G. Feletti (eds), Kogan Page, London, 1998. This contains a valuable section on assessment.

A useful practical guide to implementing PBL is **Problem Based Learning in Medicine** by T. David et al., Royal Society of Medicine Books, London, 1999.

A source of written examples of clinical problems suitable for pre-clinical and clinical courses is **Clinical Problem-Based Learning: A Workbook for Integrating Basic and Clinical Science** by R. Waterman et al., University of New Mexico Press, Albuquerque, 1988. It is also recommended that examples are sought from other PBL schools, some of which are available on the Web.

Books and articles referred to in this chapter

H. Barrows (1986). A taxonomy of problem-based learning methods. *Medical Education*, **20**, 481-6.

A. Kaufman et al. (1989). The New Mexico experiment: educational innovation and institutional change. *Academic Medicine*, **64**, 285-94.

G. Feletti and S. Carver (eds.) (1989). The new pathway to general medical education at Harvard University. *Teaching and Learning in Medicine*, **1**, 42-6.

Additional references

The following is a selection of references which will be a good starting point for someone wishing to become more informed about the research evidence for PBL.

M. Albanese (2000). Problem-based learning: why curricula are likely to show little effect on knowledge and clinical skills. *Medical Education*, **34**, 729-738.

J. Colliver (2000). Effectiveness of PBL curricula. *Academic Medicine*, **75**, 259-266.

R. Foley, A. Polson and J. Vance (1997). Review of the literature on PBL in the clinical setting. *Teaching and Learning in Medicine*, **9**, 4-9.

G. Norman and H. Schmidt (2000). Effectiveness of PBL curricula: theory practice and paper darts. *Medical Education*, **34**, 721-728.

8:   ASSESSING THE STUDENTS

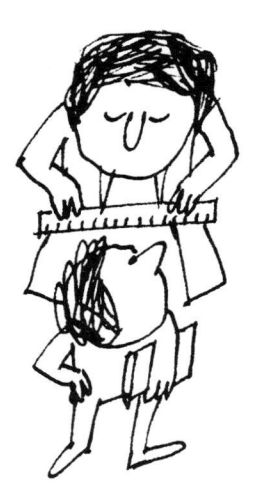

INTRODUCTION

Being involved in student assessment is among the most critical of all tasks facing the teacher. Generally, teachers take such involvement quite seriously but, sadly, the quality of many assessment and examination procedures leaves much to be desired. The aim of this chapter, therefore, will be to help you to ensure that the assessments with which you are involved do what they are supposed to do in a fair and accurate way. We will provide some background information about the purposes of assessment and the basic principles of education measurement. We will then detail the forms of assessment with which you should be familiar in order that you can select an appropriate method.

THE PURPOSE OF ASSESSMENT

When faced with developing an assessment you must be quite clear about its purpose. This may appear to be stating the obvious but try asking your colleagues and students what they think is the purpose of the assessment with which you are concerned. We are certain that there will be a considerable diversity of opinion.

Purposes of assessment may be described as follows:

- Judging mastery of essential skills and knowledge.
- Rank ordering students.
- Measuring improvement over time.
- Diagnosing student difficulties.
- Providing feedback for students.
- Evaluating the effectiveness of the course.
- Motivating students to study.
- Setting standards.
- Quality control for the public.

Though it may be possible for one assessment method to achieve more than one of these purposes, all too often assessments are used for inappropriate purposes and consequently fail to provide valid and reliable data.

It must never be forgotten how powerfully an assessment affects students, particularly if it is one on which their future may depend. This influence may be positive or negative and even harmful. For many students, passing the examination at the end of the course is their primary motivation. Should this examination not be valid, and thus not truly reflect the content and objectives of the course, then the potential for serious distortions in learning and for making errors of judgement about students is evident. An example from our own experience may illustrate this point. A revision of the final-year medical curriculum inadvertently led to the multiple-choice test component of the end-of-year assessment having considerably more weight than the clinical component. Students were observed to be spending excessive amounts of time studying the theoretical aspects of the course in preference to practising their clinical skills, the latter being the main aim of the curriculum revision. A subsequent modification of the assessment scheme, giving equal weighting to an assessment of clinical competence, corrected this unsatisfactory state of affairs.

It is our view that assessments on which decisions about the students' future are to be made (summative assessment) should be kept separate from those which are for the benefit of the students in terms of guiding their further study (formative assessment) as they have profoundly different effects on student behaviour.

Summative assessment

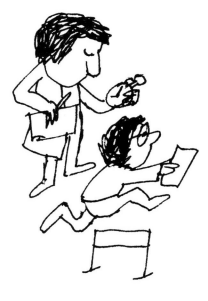

In dealing with summative assessment, every effort must be made to ensure that all assessments are fair and based on appropriate criteria. Students should be fully informed of these criteria, on the assessment methods to be employed and on the weightings to be given to each component. Such information should be given to students when a course begins. This is important because it is surprising how often information obtained from other sources, such as past students or even from the institution itself, can be inaccurate, misleading or misinterpreted by the students. The best way of avoiding this is to publish details of the course plan, including the assessment scheme. Examples of past papers can be provided and we have found an open forum on the assessment scheme early in the course to be both popular and valuable.

Formative assessment

Formative assessments are generally organised more informally and undertaken on a continuous basis. Such assessments must be free of threat, as the aim is to get the students to reveal their strengths and weaknesses rather than to disguise them – the opposite to the students' approach to summative assessments. Opportunities to obtain feedback on knowledge or performance are always appreciated by students and can lead to positive feelings about the department and the staff concerned.

WHAT YOU SHOULD KNOW ABOUT EDUCATIONAL MEASUREMENT

Whatever the purpose of the assessment, the method used should satisfy the following requirements:

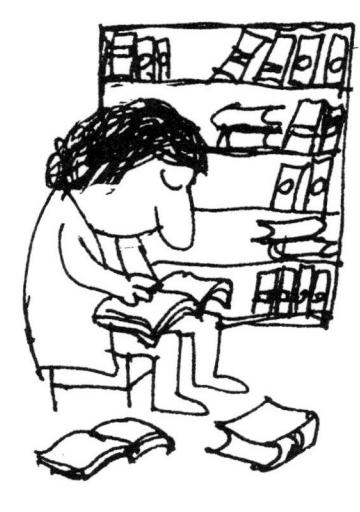

1 **Validity:** does it measure what it is supposed to measure?

2 **Reliability:** does it produce consistent results?

3 **Practicality:** Is it practical in terms of time and resources?

4 **Positive impact on learning**.

Our intention in raising these requirements is to encourage you to apply the same critical interest in the quality of educational assessment as you undoubtedly apply to the quality of the methods used in your research or patient care. This section will provide you with some basic information about the aspects of educational measurement with which we think you should be familiar.

Validity

Content validity is the first priority of any assessment. It is a measure of the degree to which the assessment contains a representative sample of the material taught in the course. A numerical value cannot be placed against it and it must be judged according to the objectives of the assessment. Therefore, in approaching any assessment the first question you must ask is: **what are the objectives of the course?**

Unfortunately, such objectives are not always available. Should you be in this situation, with no written objectives

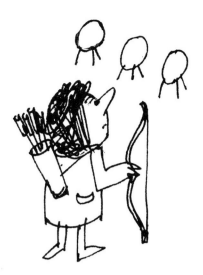

for the assessment you have to design, then you have no alternative but to develop them. This is not such a difficult task as you might imagine because, as far as the assessment is concerned, the objectives are embodied in the course content. A look at the teaching programme, lecture and tutorial topics, and discussions with teaching staff should allow you to identify and categorise the key features of the course. What you are, in fact, attempting to do is to construct a course plan in reverse and you may find it helpful at this point to consult Chapter 6 on course planning where this process is discussed in greater detail.

The objectives of the course are the blueprint against which you can evaluate the content validity. For the content validity to be high, the assessment must sample the students' abilities **on each objective**. As these objectives are likely to cover a wide range of knowledge, skills and attitudes, it will immediately become apparent that no single test method is likely to provide a valid assessment. For instance, a multiple-choice test will hardly be likely to provide valid information about clinical skills. Some objectives, particularly those in the attitudinal area will be hard to assess validly in examination settings and alternative forms of assessment may have to be sought.

Other forms of validity exist but generally speaking you will not be in a position to evaluate them so they will not be discussed further. If you are interested, you should consult the Guided Reading at the end of the chapter.

Reliability

The reliability of any assessment is a measure of the consistency and precision with which it tests what it is supposed to test. Though its importance is initially less vital than validity, you should remember that an unreliable assessment cannot be valid. The degree of reliability varies with the assessment format itself, the quality of its administration and the marking.

Theoretically, a reliable assessment should produce the same result if administered to the same student on two separate occasions. Various methods are available which provide statistical indices of reliability and you should seek expert advice on these. A common approach used in multiple-choice tests is to produce a measure of **internal consistency.**

Another key component in determining the reliability of an assessment is the **consistency of the marking**. The absence of consistency is a major reason for the unacceptable levels of reliability in most forms of direct assessment, in clinical examinations and in written tests of the essay type. However, methods are available to help you minimise this problem and these will be discussed later in this chapter.

It has become widely recognised in recent years that an even more important contributor to unreliability is inadequate content or performance sampling. This is a particular problem for assessments of clinical competence which need to be much longer than is usually the case if high levels of reliability (generalisability) are to be achieved. You must explore this issue further if you are involved in developing a 'high stakes' clinical examination such as ones to be used for certification purposes.

Improving validity and reliability of assessments

Validity can be improved by:

- carefully matching an assessment with the learning objectives, content and teaching methods;
- increasing the sample of objectives and content areas included in any assessment;
- producing an examination blueprint (see Figure 8.1);
- using test methods that are appropriate for the objectives specified;
- employing a range of test methods;
- ensuring adequate security and supervision to avoid cheating in examinations;
- improving the reliability of the assessment.

Reliability can be improved by:

- ensuring that questions are clear and suitable for the level of the students;
- checking to make sure time limits are realistic;
- writing instructions that are simple, clear, and unambiguous;
- developing a marking scheme of high quality (e.g.

FIGURE 8.1.
OUTLINE BLUEPRINT FOR A CLINICAL COMPETENCE EXAMINATION

Competence categories	Problem 1	Problem 2	Problem 3	Problem 4	Problem 5
HISTORY TAKING	X				
PHYSICAL EXAMINATION		X			
ASSESSMENT/ DIAGNOSTIC ACUMEN			X		
INVESTIGATION				X	
MANAGEMENT/TREATMENT					X
DOCTOR–PATIENT RELATIONSHIP/ COMMUNICATION SKILLS	X				

Notes: 1. Problems are patient presentations e.g. chest pain, diarrhoea, headache

2. Crosses indicate a theoretical process to ensure validity by sampling equally across competencies and problems.

explicit and agreed criteria, checking of marks, several skilled markers);

● keeping choices within a test paper to a minimum;
● when using less reliable methods increasing the number of questions, observations or examination time.

Practicality

An assessment scheme must be practical. You may decide to use a scheme that is potentially highly valid and reliable but find that it is not practical to do so in your circumstances. Some questions you might consider here are:

- Do I have the skills to administer, mark and grade the assessment?
- Can I interpret the results accurately?
- Will the assessment scheme demand too much time?
- Does the scheme require special resources (e.g. labour, materials or equipment) and are these readily available to me?
- If appropriate, can I combine less reliable methods with more reliable methods?

Obviously, there will be other considerations of a practical nature that are peculiar to your own circumstances and that you will have to consider before implementing any particular scheme.

Norm-referenced versus criterion-referenced assessment

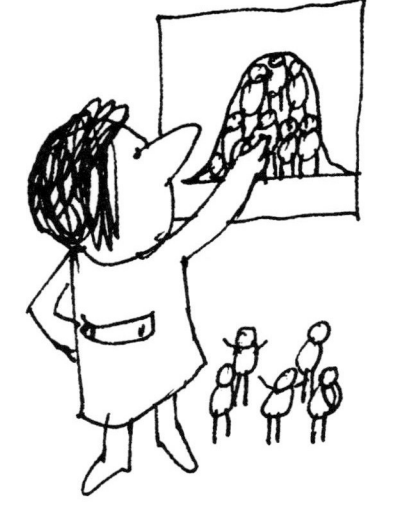

Before we finish dealing with some of the basic principles of educational measurement, we wish to introduce the difference between norm- and criterion-referenced assessment. You are likely to be familiar with norm-referenced assessment, as this reflects the traditional approach to testing. Any assessment which uses the results of all the students to determine the standard is of this type. In such tests the pass level is often set by predetermining the proportion of students given each grade or 'grading on the curve' as it is often called. This is also sometimes called a *relative* standard setting procedure.

This traditional approach is one that we urge you to move away from. Some assumptions made are not appropriate to assessing learning in universities, and the approach can be shown to lack an educational justification. For example, do we seriously set out in our teaching to ensure that, no matter how well students achieve the objectives, because of our grading on the curve policy, some will fail? Surely, our task is to help all students to achieve the objectives and reduce gaps between them rather than getting a 'spread of scores'. We refer you to Biggs to understand this concept more fully.

In medicine we are often more concerned to establish that the students achieve some minimal standard of competence. In this case, the criterion-referenced approach is more appropriate. Such an approach necessitates the determination of an **absolute** standard before administering the assessment, rather than waiting to see the overall results before doing so. Though this can be difficult to implement, we have found that attempting to do so is a powerful way of improving the validity of the assessment. Everyone concerned is forced to consider each item in the assessment and ask themselves if it is relevant and set at the appropriate level of difficulty. Our own experiences with such an approach used to test clinical competence in the final year of the medical degree have been very revealing and rewarding.

The issue of **standard setting** is one which is achieving growing attention as the focus of assessment moves from norm-referenced to criterion-referenced or competency based testing. Established procedures are available for setting absolute standards in objective-type tests but are less well developed for clinical examinations. This is too complex and too difficult an area to discuss in this book but reading the article by Norcini is strongly recommended if you have responsibility for a 'high stakes' examination.

Positive impact on learning

It is clear that how and what students learn is influenced more by our assessment practices than by any other factor in the curriculum. This influence is exerted at two levels. At a policy level, an over-emphasis on formal examinations and the implicit threat that this may carry will have a negative impact. At a methodological level, an emphasis on objective tests, such as true/false and multiple-choice, will almost certainly encourage and reward the use of surface learning strategies by students rather than approaches that demand higher-level intellectual processes such as reasoning and analysis. On the other hand, there are several assessment practices that can encourage and reward the kinds of learning that are more highly valued today. These approaches include direct assessments of performance, learning portfolios, research projects, self and peer assessment, and regular and constructive feedback on learning.

If we appreciate this influence, then we have a solution to the problem. In the criterion-referenced approach described above, the objectives are embedded in the assessment tasks, so if students focus on assessment, they will be learning what the objectives say they should be learning. This is a positive solution to the common problem of the negative impact of assessment.

ASSESSMENT METHODS

In planning your assessment, it is necessary to be aware of the variety of methods available to you. It is impossible to be comprehensive for reasons of space so we will restrict ourselves to some common methods. We will also include information about some innovative approaches developed recently, which may be of interest. We do this deliberately in an attempt to encourage you to become subversive! With your new-found knowledge of assessment you will soon be involved in situations where it is obvious that inappropriate methods are being used. This may be due to a combination of tradition, ignorance and prejudice. The first two you may be able to influence by rational argument based on the type of information we provide in this book. The last is a more difficult problem with which to deal.

TYPES OF ASSESSMENT

1 Essay
2 Short-answer
3 Structured
4 Objective tests
5 Direct observation
6 Oral
7 Structured clinical/practical assessment
8 Self-assessment
9 Learning portfolio

1. ESSAY

We suggest caution in the use of the essay, except in situations where its unique attributes are required. The essay is the only means we have to assess the students' ability to compose an answer and present it in effective

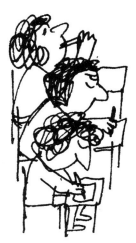

prose. It can also indirectly measure attitudes, values and opinions. There are other reasons for retaining essays for some purposes. Of particular importance in higher education seems to be the assumption that the production of written language and the expression of thought are scholarly activities of considerable worth and that essays encourage students to develop more desirable study habits.

Though they are relatively easy to set, essays are time-consuming to mark. The widespread use of multiple-choice tests and the advent of computer scoring has lifted the marking burden from many academics, few of whom would wish to take it up again. Excluding such selfish reasons, there are other grounds for being concerned about using essays. The most important is the potential for unreliable marking. Several studies have shown significant differences between the marks allocated by difference examiners and even by the same examiner re-marking the same papers at a later date.

Essay questions tend to be of two kinds. The first is the **extended response**. An example is seen in Figure 8.2.

FIGURE 8.2.
EXAMPLE OF EXTENDED
RESPONSE ESSAY QUESTION

> COMPARE AND CONTRAST ESSAY TESTS WITH
> OBJECTIVE TESTS IN MEDICAL EDUCATION

In the extended response question the student's factual knowledge and ability to provide and organise ideas, to substantiate them and to present them in coherent English are tested. The extended essay is useful for testing knowledge objectives at the higher levels such as analysis and evaluation.

Another type of essay question is the **restricted response**, an example of which is shown in Figure 8.3. The restricted response form sets boundaries on the answer required and on its organisation.

FIGURE 8.3.
EXAMPLE OF RESTRICTED
RESPONSE ESSAY QUESTION

> KIDNEY DISEASE IS A SIGNIFICANT CAUSE OF
> HYPERTENSION. DESCRIBE THE MECHANISMS BY
> WHICH THIS OCCURS

This type of essay is best for testing lower-level knowledge objectives. An advantage of the more restricted format is that it can decrease the scoring problems (and hence be more reliable).

If you intend to set and mark essay questions in an examination, then we suggest that you keep in mind the points in Figure 8.4.

For essays, or other written assignments required during a course of study, you should take steps to improve the quality of feedback to students. One way is to use a structured assignment attachment. Not only can such an attachment provide very useful individual feedback, but used early in a course with a model answer, it can show students the standards you expect from them, and also help you in awarding marks.

2. SHORT-ANSWER AND SIMPLE COMPUTATION QUESTIONS

Short-answer tests have been surprisingly little used in recent years, yet another casualty of the multiple-choice boom. However, we have found them increasingly useful as our concerns about the limitations of the objective type tests have become more apparent.

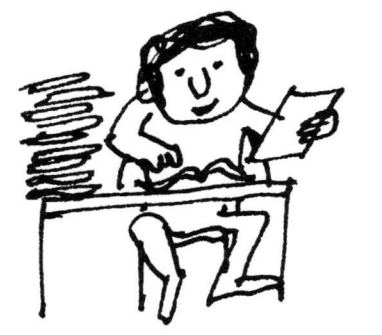

Though easy to mark, it is essential that markers are provided with a well constructed marking key, especially if more than one correct answer is possible, or if several processes are involved in answering the question (See Figure 8.5).

Obviously more short-answer questions than essays can be fitted into a fixed time period. If one of the purposes of the assessment is to cover a wide content area, then short-answer questions have distinct advantages. Much of the same may be said about multiple-choice questions but short-answer questions have the advantage of avoiding cueing and requiring students to supply an answer, rather than to select or to guess from a fixed number of options. The major limitation of the short-answer test is that it is not suitable for testing complex learning outcomes.

If you wish to employ short-answer questions you should take account of the point in Figure 8.6.

FIGURE 8.4.
PROCEDURE FOR SETTING
AND MARKING ESSAY
QUESTIONS

Procedure

A Write questions that elicit the type of response suggested by the objectives

Use clear directive words such as 'describe', 'compare', 'contrast', 'criticize' and 'explain'. If 'discuss' is used, be sure to indicate what points should be discussed.

Establish a clear framework which aims the student to the desired response. Rather than: 'Discuss beta-blockers', try 'Describe the benefits and potential hazards of beta-blockers in the treatment of heart disease'.

B Set a relatively large number of questions requiring short answers of about a page rather than a few questions requiring long answers of three or four pages

This will provide a better sampling of course content and you will reduce bias in marking for quantity rather than quality.

C Ensure that all students are required to answer the same questions

Constructing optional questions of equal difficulty is hard and, further, you will not be able to make valid comparisons among students if they have answered different questions.

D Prepare a marking system

Two methods are commonly used, both of which require you to prepare a model answer. In the analytical method of marking, a checklist of specific points is prepared against which marks are allocated. Such factors as 'logical argument' or 'expression' should be included if you think they are relevant. If you wish to reward legibility and presentation give these components a proportion of the marks but avoid these aspects unduly biasing your assessment of the content. The global method of marking can be used if you have at least 30 papers to mark. Papers are read rapidly and assigned to one of five or more piles, grading from a superior response down to the inferior. Papers are then re-read to check the original sorting. This is a faster and more reliable method of marking once standards for the various piles have been established.

E Mark questions with the following points in mind

Mark anonymously.

Mark only one question at a time or, preferably, have a separate marker for each question.

Adopt consistent standards.

Try to mark one question without interruption.

Re-read a sample of papers to check marking consistency.

F Prepare feedback

As you mark keep in mind that one of the most powerful influences on learning is the quality of feedback provided to students. Keep a record of issues for individuals or group feedback.

FIGURE 8.5.
EXAMPLES OF SIMPLE
SHORT-ANSWER QUESTIONS
WITH ANSWER KEYS

> AN ELDERLY PATIENT PRESENTS WITH A TREMOR WHICH IS PRESENT AT REST, MADE WORSE BY ANXIETY AND DECREASED WITH INTENTION. YOU NOTE THAT THIS IS NOT PRESENT WHEN THE PATIENT IS ASLEEP. WHAT IS THE LIKELY DIAGNOSIS
>
> **ANSWER:** PARKINSONISM (1 MARK)

> A SERUM BIOCHEMICAL SCREEN REVEALS A LOW CALCIUM, A LOW PHOSPHATE AND A RAISED ALKALINE PHOSPHATASE. LIST TWO TYPICAL SYMPTOMS YOU WOULD EXPECT THIS PATIENT TO HAVE
>
> **ANSWER:** BONE PAIN; MUSCLE WEAKNESS; DIFFICULTY IN WALKING (1 MARK FOR TWO CORRECT ANSWERS; 1/2 MARK FOR ONE CORRECT ANSWER)

FIGURE 8.6.
PROCEDURE FOR SETTING
AND MARKING SHORT-
ANSWER QUESTIONS

> **Procedure**
>
> **A** Make the questions precise
>
> **B** Prepare a structured marking sheet
> Allocate marks or part marks for the acceptable answer(s).
> Be prepared to consider other equally acceptable answers, some of which you may not have predicted.
>
> **C** Mark questions with the following points in mind
> Mark anonymously.
> Complete the marking of one page of questions at a time.
> Preferably have a different examiner for each page of questions to reduce bias.

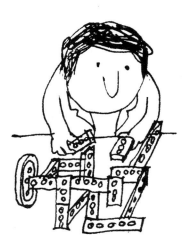

3. STRUCTURED TESTS

Broadly speaking there are two types of structured tests which are used in medical education – patient management problems (PMPs) and modified essay questions (MEQs). Both claim to assess problem-solving skills.

Patient management problems

PMPs aim to represent, with varying degrees of fidelity, an interaction with a patient incorporating various amounts of data gathering, diagnosis and management. Written formats, using many ingenious technical devices, were quite widely used at one stage particularly in postgraduate education. However, difficulties with developing valid scoring systems have led to a marked reduction in their use and it seems unlikely that many medical school teachers will be called on to develop them.

On the other hand the use of computer-based PMPs is a rapidly expanding field particularly in North America where they are increasingly being used in national certifying examinations. The levels of expertise required to construct these sophisticated simulations are beyond those expected of the average medical teacher so will not be considered further in this book. However, we strongly recommend looking at examples of such PMPs which are available on the Web, and consider incorporating them into teaching programmes. Good quality versions will be popular with your students.

Modified essay questions

This test was initially developed for the Royal College of General Practitioners in London. The MEQ is now being used with increasing frequency. The term essay is perhaps a little misleading because the format more closely resembles a series of short-answer questions than an essay.

The student is provided with a limited amount of patient data and then asked to write a brief answer to a question. Such questions may relate to history taking, examination findings, diagnosis, investigations and so on. Following one or more initial questions, further information may be provided and additional questions posed.

A certain amount of skill is required when preparing an MEQ to avoid giving the answers to previous questions and to avoid the student being repeatedly penalised for the same error. Scoring is by comparison of the student's answer with model answers. The precautions to be taken in marking are the same as those described for marking short-answer questions.

MEQs are very popular with students, particularly when used in formative assessment. Marked papers can be returned or the students can be given the model answer and mark their own. The value of this exercise is enhanced when a tutorial is held to discuss disputes with the model answer. Their increasing use in summative assessment is probably due to the fact that when skilfully prepared it is possible to test a range of disciplinary aspects within the one question, a major advantage as examinations become more integrated.

An example of an MEQ is seen in Figure 8.7.

4. OBJECTIVE TESTS

This generic term is used in education to include a variety of test formats in which the marking of the answers is objective. Some classifications include short-answer questions in this category. The term multiple-choice test is sometimes used synonymously with the term objective test. However, we encourage you to use the more general term 'objective tests' as it allows us to include a wide variety of test types, only one of which can be accurately described as 'multiple-choice'. Other commonly used examples of objective tests are the true-false and matching types.

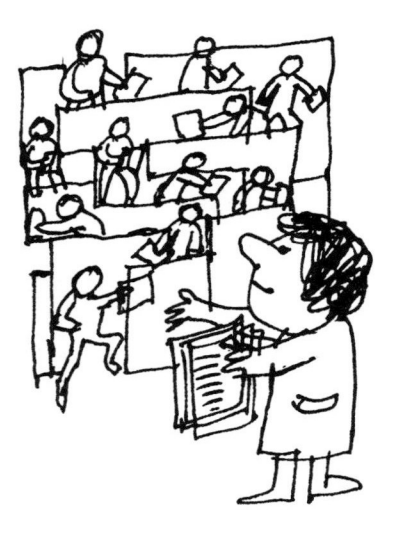

The characteristics of such tests are the high reliability of the scoring, the rapidity of scoring and the economy of staff time in this task, and the ability to test large content areas. They lend themselves to the development of banks of questions, thus further reducing the time of examination preparation in the long-term. These advantages have sometimes led to an over-reliance on objective tests and a failure to be critical in their use.

While it is relatively easy to write objective items to measure the recall of bits of factual knowledge, consider-

FIGURE 8.7.
EXAMPLE OF THE START OF A
MODIFIED ESSAY QUESTION

Please answer all the questions in sequence. Do **not** look through the book before you start.

Mr Smith, a 78-year-old widower who lives alone, complains of lethargy and weight loss. He has been admitted to the general medical unit on which you work for further investigation.

Q1   What are the three most likely diagnoses?

    a.

    b.

    c

Q2   List five specific questions which would help you distinguish between these possibilities.

    a.

    b.

    c.

    d.

    e.

A routine blood test ordered by his general practitioner reveals a haemoglobin of 10.4 g/dl and the anaemia is reported to be of the microcytic hypochromic type.

Q3   List two typical clinical signs you would look for when you examine the patient.

    a.

    b.

Q4   Briefly describe how this information has affected your first diagnosis.

able skill is required to write items that measure higher-level intellectual skills.

While it is possible you will not have to set and mark other forms of written test, it is almost certain that you will have to participate in some way in writing or administering objective tests.

Choosing the type of question

You must find out or decide which type of item you will be using. Objective items can be classified into three groups: **true-false, multiple-choice** and **matching**. We would suggest you avoid the more complex matching types which, in some examinations, often seem to behave more like tests of reading ability, rather then tests of the course content! For a variety of technical reasons, experts favour multiple-choice over true-false and other types of objective items.

True-false questions

Examples of true-false questions are shown in Figures 8.8 and 8.9.

FIGURE 8.8.
EXAMPLE OF SIMPLE TRUE-FALSE ITEM

Ⓣ F   IN A 40-YEAR-OLD PATIENT WITH MILD HYPERTENSION YOU WOULD CONSIDER COMMENCING TREATMENT WITH ATENOLOL

FIGURE 8.9.
EXAMPLE OF MULTIPLE (CLUSTER) TRUE-FALSE ITEM

IN A 40-YEAR-OLD PATIENT WITH MILD HYPERTENSION YOU WOULD CONSIDER COMMENCING TREATMENT WITH

Ⓣ F   ATENOLOL
T Ⓕ   HYDRALAZINE
Ⓣ F   BENDROFLUAZIDE
Ⓣ F   NIFEDIPINE
T Ⓕ   AMILORIDE

The **simple type** will obviously cause you the least problems in construction and scoring. The more complex **multiple type** (also know as the cluster type) is very popular because it allows a series of questions to be asked relating to a single stem or topic. Each question may be marked as a separate question. However, the questions may also be considered as a group with full marks given only if all the questions are correct and part-marks given if varying proportions of the questions are correct. Research has shown that the ranking of students is unaltered by the marking scheme used, so simplicity should be the guiding principle.

If you intend to use true-false questions you should take particular note of the points listed in Figure 8.10.

FIG 8.10.
PROCEDURE FOR SETTING TRUE-
FALSE QUESTIONS

Procedure

A Make sure the content of the question is important and relevant and that the standard is appropriate to the group being tested.

B Use statements which are short, unambiguous and contain only one idea.

C Ensure the statement is indeed unequivocally true or false.

D Avoid words which are giveaways to the correct answer, such as sometimes, always or never.

E Make sure true statements and false statements are the same length and are written in approximately equal numbers.

F Avoid negative or double-negative statements.

Multiple-choice questions

An example of a simple multiple-choice question (MCQ) is shown in Figure 8.11.

FIG 8.11.
EXAMPLE OF A SIMPLE
MULTIPLE-CHOICE ITEM

IN A 40-YEAR-OLD PATIENT WITH MILD HYPERTENSION WHICH ONE OF THE FOLLOWING WOULD YOU USE TO COMMENCE TREATMENT?

1. ATENOLOL
2. HYDRALAZINE
3. CLONIDINE
4. AMILORIDE
5. METHYL DOPA

The MCQ illustrated is made up of a stem ('In a 40 year old') and five alternative answers. Of these alternatives one is correct and the others are known as 'distractors'.

One advantage of the MCQ over the true-false question is a reduction in the influence of guessing. Obviously, in a simple true-false question there is a 50 per cent chance of guessing the correct answer. In a one from five MCQ there is only a 20 per cent chance of doing so if all the distractors are working effectively. Unfortunately it is hard to achieve this ideal and exam-wise students may easily be able to eliminate one or two distractors and thus reduce the number of options from which they have to guess. Information about the effectiveness of the distractors is usually available after the examination if it has been computer-marked. Some advocate the use of correction formulas for guessing but this does not – on balance – appear to be worth the effort and may add an additional student-related bias to the results.

If you intend to use multiple-choice questions you should take particular note of the points in Figure 8.12.

FIGURE 8.12.
PROCEDURE FOR SETTING
MULTIPLE-CHOICE QUESITONS

Procedure

A Make sure the content of the question is important and relevant and that the standard is appropriate to the group being tested.

B The main content of the question should be in the stem and the alternatives should be kept as short as possible.

C Eliminate redundant information from the stem (this fault often applies to clinical items containing patient data).

D Ensure each distractor is a plausible answer which cannot be eliminated from consideration because it is irrelevant or silly.

E Avoid giving clues to correct or incorrect responses which have nothing to do with the content of the question.

- Make sure correct and incorrect responses are of similar length.
- Check the grammar, particularly when the alternative is written as the completion of a statement in the stem.
- Distribute the place of the correct response equally among positions 1 to 5 (or 1 to 4 as the case may be).

F Do not use an 'all of the above' or 'none of the above' alternative.

G Avoid negatives.

H Do not write trick questions.

Context-dependent questions

Having mastered the basic principles of setting good objective items, you may wish to become more adventurous. It is possible to develop questions with a more complex stem which may require a degree of analysis before the answer is chosen. Such items are sometimes known as context-dependent multiple-choice questions.

One or more multiple-choice questions are based on stimulus material which may be presented in the form of a clinical scenario, a diagram, a graph, a table of data, a statement from a text or research report, a photograph and so on. This approach is useful if one wishes to attempt to test the student's ability at a higher intellectual level than simple recognition and recall of factual information.

Extended-matching questions

The technical limitations of conventional objective-type items for use in medical examinations has stimulated a search for alternative forms which retain the technical advantages of computer scoring. Many such efforts have achieved little more than increasing complexity and confusion for students. However, the extended matching question (EMQ) is becoming increasingly popular. The main technical advantage is the reduced impact of cueing by increasing the number of distractors. Other advantages include ease of construction and flexibility as they work equally well for basic science as for clinical areas. However, they are particularly well suited for testing diagnostic and management skills. An example of an EMQ is given in Figure 8.13.

The EMQ is typically made up of four parts: a theme of related concepts; a list of options; a lead-in statement to direct students; and two or more item stems.

The item shown includes two stems that illustrate how this EMQ might test at different levels. The first stem requires problem solving in order to determine a diagnosis; the second stem tests only recall. More stems could, of course, be added to this example to increase the content coverage of the test item and the range of levels tested. In some respects, EMQs share similarities with the context-dependent MCQ we described earlier.

FIGURE 8.13.
EXAMPLE OF AN EXTENDED-MATCHING QUESTON (ADAPTED FROM CASE AND SWANSON)

THEME: **METABOLIC ABNORMALITIES**

OPTIONS: A.   VITAMIN A   I.   BIOTIN
           B.   VITAMIN B1   J.   COPPER
           C.   VITAMIN B2   K.   FOLATE
           D.   VITAMIN B6   L.   IODINE
           E.   VITAMIN C   M.   IRON
           F.   VITAMIN D   N.   MAGNESIUM
           G.   VITAMIN E   O.   NIACIN
           H.   VITAMIN K   P.   ZINC

LEAD-IN: FOR EACH PATIENT WITH CLINICAL FEATURES CAUSED BY METABOLIC ABNORMALITIES,
           SELECT THE VITAMIN OR MINERAL THAT IS MOST LIKELY TO BE INVOLVED.

STEMS: **1.**   A 70-YEAR-OLD WIDOWER HAS ECCHYMOSES, PERIFOLLICULAR
                   PETECHIAE, AND SWELLING OF THE GINGIVA. HIS DIET CONSISTS OF
                   COLA AND HOT DOGS.
                   (ANSWER: E)

         2.   INVOLVED IN CLOTTING FACTOR SYNTHESIS.
                   (ANSWER: H)

Putting together an objective test

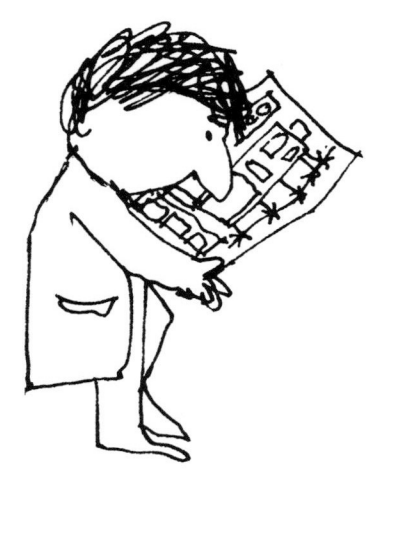

This is the point where many tests come to grief. It is not enough simply to select 100 questions from the item bank or from among those recently prepared by your colleagues. The selection must be done with great care and must be based on the objectives of the course. A **blueprint**, or table of test specifications, should be prepared which identifies the key topics of the course which must be tested. The number of questions to be allocated to each topic should then be determined according to its relative importance. Once this is done the job becomes easier. Sort out the items into the topics and select those which cover as many areas within the topic as possible. It is advisable to have a small working group at this stage to check the quality of the questions and to avoid your personal bias in the selection process. You may find that there are some topics for which there is an inadequate number or variety of questions. You should then commission the writing of additional items from appropriate colleagues or, if time is short, your committee may have to undertake this task. This process of blue-printing will establish the content validity of the test.

The questions should now be put in order. It is less confusing to students if the items for each topic are kept together. Check to see that the correct answers are randomly distributed throughout the paper and if not, reorder accordingly. Organise for the paper to be word-processed, with suitable instructions about the format required and the need for security. At the same time make sure that the 'Instructions to Students' section at the beginning of the paper is clear and accurate. Check and recheck the copy as errors are almost invariably discovered during the examination, a cause of much consternation. Finally, have the paper printed and arrange for secure storage until the time of the examination.

Scoring and analysing an objective test

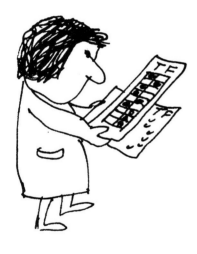

The main advantage of the objective type tests is the rapidity with which scoring can be done. This requires some attention to the manner in which the students are to answer the questions. It is usually inappropriate to have the students mark their answers on the paper itself. When large numbers are involved a separate structured sheet should be used. Where facilities are available it is convenient to use answer sheets that can be directly scored by computer or for responses to be entered directly into a computer by students. However, a hand-marking answer sheet can easily be prepared. An overlay is produced by cutting out the positions of the correct responses. This can then be placed over the student's answer sheet and the correct responses are easily and rapidly counted. Before doing so ensure that the student has not marked more than one answer correct!

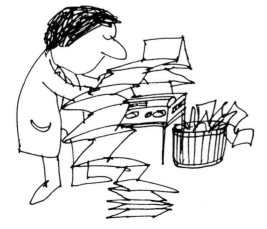

In most major medical examinations a computer will be used to score and analyse objective-type examinations. You must therefore be familiar with the process and be able to interpret the subsequent results. The computer programme will generally provide statistical data about the examination including a reliability coefficient for internal consistency, a mean and standard deviation for the class and analyses of individual items. Should you be the person responsible for the examination you will need to know how to interpret this information in order to process the examination results and to help improve subsequent examinations. If you are not familiar with these aspects we strongly suggest you seek expert advice or consult one of the books on educational measurement listed at the end of the chapter.

5. DIRECT OBSERVATION

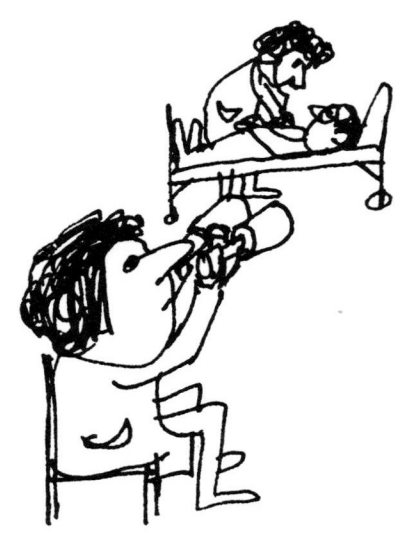

Direct observation of the student performing a technical or an interpersonal skill in the real, simulated or examination setting would appear to be the most valid way of assessing such skills. Unfortunately, the reliability of these observations is likely to be seriously low. This is particularly so in the complex interpersonal area where no alternative form of assessment is available. Nevertheless, in professional courses it is essential to continue to make assessments of the student's performance, not least to indicate to the student your commitment to these vital skills. In doing so, you would be well advised to use the information predominantly for feedback rather than for important decision-making.

Various ways have been suggested by which these limitations might be minimised. One it to improve the method of scoring and another is to improve the performance of the observer. The former involves the design of checklists and ratings forms.

Checklists

A checklist is basically a two-point rating scale. Evidence suggests that the reliability of a checklist decreases when there are more than four points on the scale. The assessor has to decide whether each component on the list is present/absent; adequate/inadequate; satisfactory/unsatisfactory. Only if each component is very clearly defined and readily observable can a checklist be reliable. They are particularly useful for assessing technical skills.

An example is shown in Figure 8.14.

FIGURE 8.14.
EXAMPLE OF A CLINICAL SKILLS
CHECKLIST

Examiner's instructions to students
This patient presents with symptoms suggestive of intermittent claudication. Please examine the lower limbs from the cardiovascular point of view. Provide a commentary on what you are doing and what you have found.

	Adequate	*Inadequate*	*Not performed*
1 Inspection (observes and comments on skin and colour changes)			
2 Palpation: a. Temperature b. Popliteal pulse c. Post. tibial pulse d. D. pedis pulse			
3 Circulation: a. Leg elevation b. Leg dependency			
4 Auscultation (femoral)			

Rating forms

Rating forms come in many styles. The essential feature is that the observer is required to make a judgement along a scale which may be continuous or intermittent. They are widely used to assess behaviour or performance because no other methods are usually available, but the subjectivity of the assessment is an unavoidable problem. Because of this, multiple independent ratings of the same student undertaking the same activity are essential if any sort of justice is to be done. The examples in Figure 8.15 show several alternative structures for rating the same ability. They are derived from published formats used to obtain information about ward performance of trainee doctors. The component skill being assessed is 'Obtaining the data base' and only one sub-component (obtaining information from the patient) is illustrated.

FIGURE 8.15.
EXAMPLE OF RATING FORMS

Format 1

	Top Quarter	Upper Middle Quarter	Lower Middle Quarter	Bottom Quarter
Obtaining information from the patient	4	3	2	1

Format 2

Obtaining information from the patient

☐   ☐   ☐   ☐   ☐

very effective   effective   reasonable   poor   inadequate

☐ unable to judge

Format 3

Obtaining information from the patient

Little or no information obtained	Some information obtained. Major errors or omissions	Adequate performance. Most information elicited	Very thorough exploration of patient's problems
☐	☐	☐	☐

Format 3 is the one we would recommend for two reasons. The first is that there is an attempt to provide descriptive anchor points which may be helpful in clarifying for the observer what standards should be applied. The second is a more pragmatic one. In a study we undertook, it was the format most frequently preferred by experienced clinical raters.

Improving the performance of the observer

It has often been claimed that training of raters will improve reliability. This seems to make sense but what evidence there is shows that training makes remarkably little difference! A study of our own suggested that a better approach might be to select raters who are inherently more consistent than others. Common sense dictates that observers should be adequately briefed on the ratings form and that they should not be asked to rate aspects of the student's performance that they have not observed.

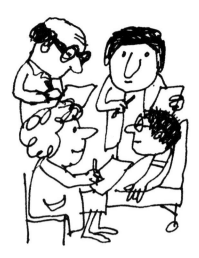

6. ORAL

The oral or vice-voce examination has for centuries been the predominant method, and sometimes the only method, used for the clinical assessment of medical students. The traditional oral, which gives considerable freedom to the examiner to vary the questions asked from student to student and to exercise personal bias, has consistently been shown to be very unreliable. One major study of traditional clinical examinations showed that the correlation between different examiners was overall no greater than would have occurred by chance!

Without doubt, face-to-face interaction between student and examiner provides a unique opportunity to test interactive skills which cannot be assessed in any other way. However, these skills are not usually the focus of attention and several studies have shown that the majority of questions in oral examinations require little more than the recall of isolated fragments of information, something more easily and more reliably assessed by more objective tests.

We would recommend that reliance on traditional oral examination be considerably reduced as it is now usually possible to incorporate many of the activities currently assessed in such examinations into the objective-structured approach discussed in the next section.

Should you wish to retain oral examinations then certain steps should be undertaken to minimise the likely problems, as outlined in Figure 8.16.

7. STRUCTURED CLINICAL/PRACTICAL ASSESSMENT

In recent years there has been a search for new approaches to assessment. One of the most interesting of these developments has been the 'objective structured clinical examination' (OSCE) first described by Harden and his colleagues in Dundee and subsequently developed by ourselves and others as an integral part of our examination procedures. This approach to the assessment of clinical and practical skills has now been taken up by most medical schools and many professional bodies.

FIGURE 8.16.
PROCEDURE FOR CONDUCTING
ORAL EXAMINATIONS

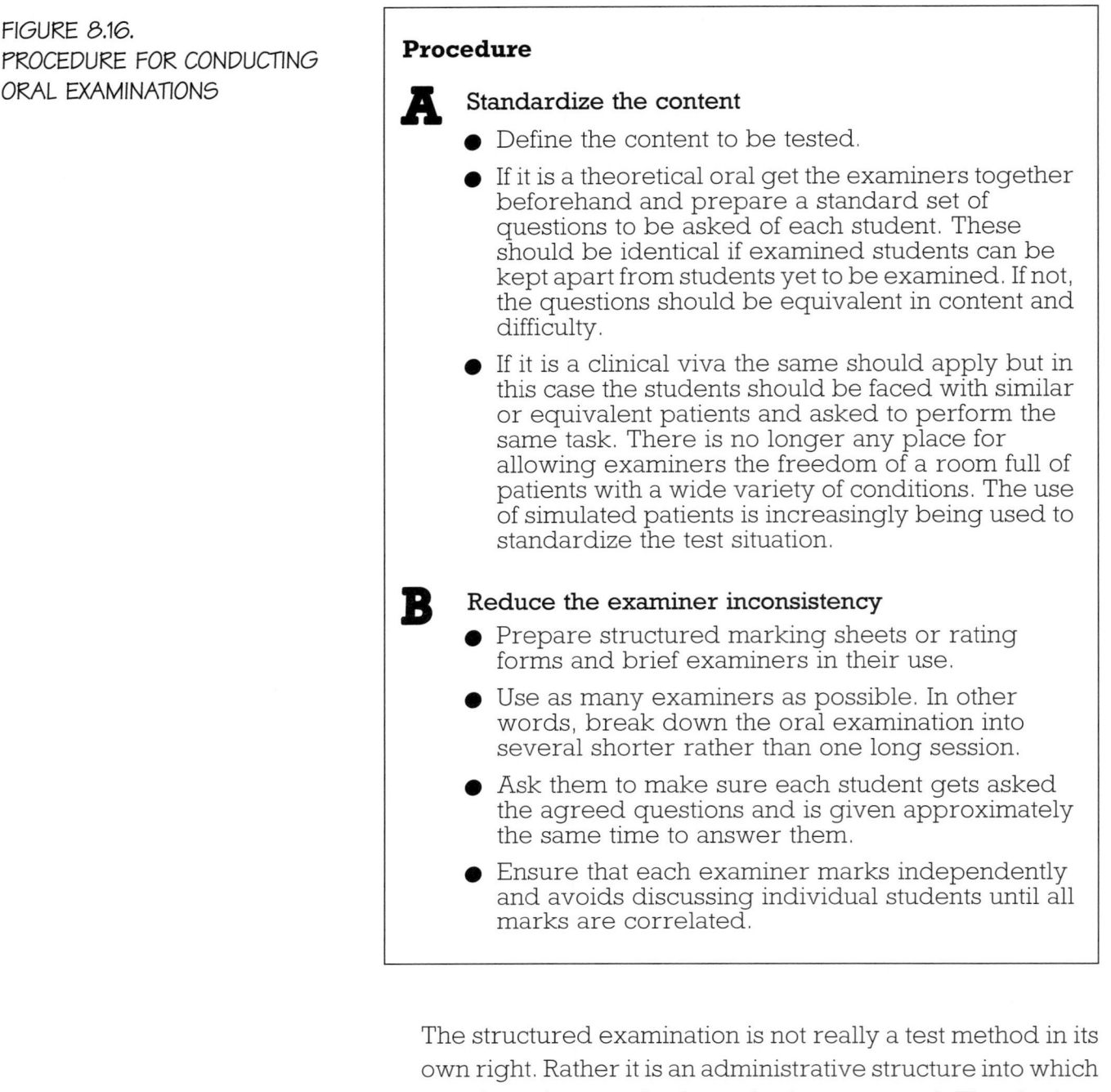

Procedure

A Standardize the content

- Define the content to be tested.

- If it is a theoretical oral get the examiners together beforehand and prepare a standard set of questions to be asked of each student. These should be identical if examined students can be kept apart from students yet to be examined. If not, the questions should be equivalent in content and difficulty.

- If it is a clinical viva the same should apply but in this case the students should be faced with similar or equivalent patients and asked to perform the same task. There is no longer any place for allowing examiners the freedom of a room full of patients with a wide variety of conditions. The use of simulated patients is increasingly being used to standardize the test situation.

B Reduce the examiner inconsistency

- Prepare structured marking sheets or rating forms and brief examiners in their use.

- Use as many examiners as possible. In other words, break down the oral examination into several shorter rather than one long session.

- Ask them to make sure each student gets asked the agreed questions and is given approximately the same time to answer them.

- Ensure that each examiner marks independently and avoids discussing individual students until all marks are correlated.

The structured examination is not really a test method in its own right. Rather it is an administrative structure into which a variety of test methods can be incorporated. The aim is to test a wide range of skills in an objective fashion.

The students proceed through a series of 'stations' and undertake a variety of tasks. Marking sheets and checklists are prepared beforehand to improve the reliability of scoring. All students are thus examined on the same content and marked on the same criteria by the same examiners. As in any form of assessment, the definition of the content to be tested, the construction of a blueprint and the preparation of good test items is essential if a high degree of validity is to be obtained. If reliability is a priority the examination will have to be a long one – probably 20-30 stations.

Figure 8.17 shows the outline of a structured clinical examination. The range of tasks to be tested is shown in the left-hand column. In the middle column is the type of assessment used which in this case includes direct observations of performance on real patients and simulators and the use of short-answer questions. The right hand column lists the time allocated to each station which in this instance is usually five minutes. However, the time allocated varies widely between different examinations used for different purposes. The advantage of short stations is that more tasks can be assessed in a given time giving cost-benefit advantages in terms of reliability.

Figure 8.18 provides an example of a structured marking sheet for a physical examination station.

Should you wish to consider introducing such an approach you should read the articles given in the references. Observation of a well run OSCE and advice from an experienced OSCE organiser will pay enormous dividends.

8. SELF-ASSESSMENT

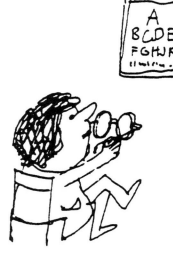

By 'self-assessment' we mean an assessment system which involves the students in establishing the criteria and standards they will apply to their work and then in making judgements about the degree to which they have been met. We believe that the skill of being able to make realistic evaluations of the quality of one's work is an attribute that every graduate should have. Yet, in conventional courses, few opportunities are provided for self-assessment skills to be learnt and developed.

The introduction of self-assessment practices into existing courses have been shown to be feasible and desirable. Whether marks generated in this way should count towards a final grade is an undecided issue. Work reported in the literature suggests that so long as the assessment scheme is well designed and students grade themselves on achievement (and not effort), they will generate marks which are reasonably consistent with staff marks. Thus, there is little doubt that self-assessment, used primarily to improve the students' understanding of their own ability and performance, is worthwhile educationally

FIGURE 8.17.
OUTLINE OF STRUCTURED CLINICAL EXAMINATION

STATION	TASK	TYPE OF ASSESSMENT	TIME (MIN)
1	ASSESSMENT OF HYPERTENSIVE PATIENT	DIRECT OBSERVATION WITH CHECK-LIST ON SIMULATED PATIENTS	10
2	COUNSELLING ON MALIGNANT BREAST LUMP	PREPATORY STATION	5
3	COUNSELLING ON MALIGNANT BREAST LUMP	DIRECT OBSERVATION WITH CHECK-LIST ON STANDARDIZED PATIENT	5
4	INTERPRETATION OF X-RAY	SHORT-ANSWER QUESTIONS	5
5	DEMONSTRATING HOW TO PERFORM A LUMBAR PUNCTURE	DIRECT OBSERVATION WITH CHECK-LIST ON SIMULATED PATIENT	5
6	EXAMINATION OF HANDS	DIRECT OBSERVATION WITH CHECK-LIST ON PATIENT WITH RHEUMATOID ARTHRITIS	5
7	REST		5
8	INTERPRETATION OF AUDIOGRAM	SHORT-ANSWER QUESTIONS	5
9	HISTORY TAKING FOR ASTHMA	DIRECT OBSERVATION WITH CHECK-LIST USING STANDARDIZED PATIENT	5
10	OPHTHALMOSCOPY IN PATIENT WITH CATARACT	DIRECT OBSERVATION WITH CHECK-LIST ON REAL PATIENT	5
11	INTERPRETATION OF CT SCAN	SHORT-ANSWER QUESTIONS	5
12	DEMONSTRATING BLOOD GLUCOSE TESTING	DIRECT OBSERVATION WITH CHECK-LIST USING SIMULATED PATIENT	5
13	PERFORMING CPR	DIRECT OBSERVATION USING CHECK-LIST ON MANIKIN	5
14	EXAMINATION OF NECK IN SUSPECTED THYROID DISEASE	DIRECT OBSERVATION USING CHECK-LIST ON REAL PATIENT	5
15	REST		5

FIGURE 8.18.
EXAMPLE OF CHECKLIST

SHORT PHYSICAL EXAMINATION – KNEE

(5 MINUTES ALLOWED)

STUDENT'S NAME:

GREET THE STUDENT AND GIVE HIM/HER THE FOLLOWING INSTRUCTIONS:

"THIS PATIENT PRESENTS WITH A HISTORY OF THE RIGHT KNEE GIVING WAY AFTER WHICH IT SWELLS. PLEASE EXAMINE THE KNEE. I WOULD LIKE YOU TO PROVIDE A COMMENTARY ON WHAT YOU ARE DOING AND WHAT YOU HAVE FOUND."

PLEASE RATE THE STUDENT ON EACH OF THE FOLLOWING CRITERIA. THE EXPECTED LEVEL OF PERFORMANCE IS THAT OF A HOSPITAL INTERN ABOUT TO COMMENCE DUTY. CIRCLE ONLY ONE MARK FOR EACH CRITERIA.

		PERFORMED ADEQUATELY AND COMPLETELY	ATTEMPTED BUT INADEQUATE OR INCOMPLETE
1	GENERAL APPROACH TO THE PATIENT (ENSURES COMFORT, IS COURTEOUS ETC)	1.00	0.50
2	INSPECTION: FOR DEFORMITY AND SWELLING, MUSCLES FOR WASTING	1.00	0.50
3	PALPATION:		
	A. CONTOURS	0.50	0.25
	B. FOR INFLAMMATION	0.50	0.25
	C. TENDERNESS (ALONG COLLATERALS AND ALONG JOINT LINE)	0.50	0.25
	D. PATELLA	0.50	0.25
	E. FLUID (MASSAGE BULGE TEST OR PATELLAR TAP)	1.00	0.50
4	MOVEMENT:		
	A. ACTIVE (BOTH KNEES)	0.50	0.25
	B. PASSIVE (BOTH KNEES)	0.50	0.25
	C. PALPATION FOR CREPITUS	0.50	0.25
5	TESTS OF STABILITY:		
	A. COLLATERAL LIGAMENTS	0.50	0.25
	B. CRUCIATE LIGAMENTS	0.50	0.25

TOTAL   SIGNED: . . . .

EXAMINER

and encourages openness and honesty about the assessment.

If you wish to embark on a trial scheme you must first set about the task of establishing criteria and standards. This can be done at a series of small group meetings attended by staff and students. Both must agree on the criteria to be applied to the students' work. To help focus on this task you might have students reflect on questions such as:

● How would you distinguish good from inadequate work?
● What would characterise a good assignment in this course?

Once criteria have been specified, students use them to judge their own performance. Marks are awarded with reference to each criterion and a statement justifying the mark should be included. An alternative is to contrast their own mark with one given to them by a peer. The teacher may also mark a random sample to establish controls and to discourage cheating or self-delusion. We urge you to give this approach to assessment very serious consideration indeed. In our view, it is among the most educationally promising ideas in recent years, and we suggest you study the book by Boud listed at the end of this chapter.

9. THE LEARNING PORTFOLIO

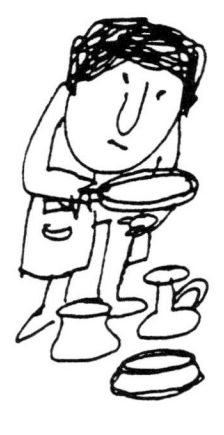

All assessment methods require that students present evidence of their learning, yet in most cases (with theses and project work being notable exceptions) it is the teacher who controls the character of that evidence. Requiring students to respond to objective tests, write essays and participate in clinical examinations for example, does this.

If we really believe in student-centred learning then we must work hard to ensure that our assessment practices reflect, encourage and reward this belief. In Chapter 1, we noted that assessment in student-centred learning needs to be more flexible with greater emphasis on student responsibility. The learning portfolio is one way of reinforcing student-centred learning. The portfolio clearly has validity as an assessment method in this situation, but its reliability for summative purposes has yet to be determined. This should not, however, discourage you from experimenting with learning portfolios with your students.

A learning portfolio is a collection of evidence presented by students to demonstrate what learning has taken place. In the portfolio, the student assembles, presents, explains, and evaluates his or her learning in relation to the objectives of the course and his or her own purposes and goals. Used for many years in disciplines like the fine arts and architecture, portfolios are now being used more widely and are being strongly advocated as an approach to the revalidation (re-certification) of practising doctors in the UK. They also have particular relevance in problem-based learning.

A learning portfolio might have several parts, such as:

- An introductory statement defining what the objectives are and what the student hopes to accomplish.
- A presentation of items of evidence to show what learning has taken place.
- An explanation of why items are chosen and presented, evidence of the application of learning to some issue or real-life situation, and an evaluation of learning outcomes.

A danger of using portfolios is that students might do too much, and some of their material might be less than relevant! So it is important to provide structure and to suggest sample items, the number of different items and their approximate size. Obviously, the items in a portfolio will reflect your particular discipline. Some ideas are listed in Figure 8.19.

Implementing learning portfolios as an assessment method requires careful preparation and planning on your part. In his discussion of portfolios, Biggs recommends that most of the following should be considered, and we suggest you look at his book for more information on these matters:

- Clarify for students, perhaps in the course objectives, what the evidence for good learning might be;
- Specify the requirements for a learning portfolio in terms of:

FIGURE 8.19.
POSSIBLE CONTENT FOR A
LEARNING PORTFOLIO

- A brief report of a student research project or other learning activity carried out individually or with peers.
- Answers to some objective test items or problems, giving both the answer and an explanation as to why the answer is correct, and possibly comments on the test items themselves.
- An abstract of a book or journal article with an explanation as to why the reading was considered important.
- A taped interview with a patient.
- A description of how materials and resources were used in learning (eg. texts, libraries, other people, and the Internet etc).
- An account of involvement in an activity, student association or society and how that involvement assisted with learning.
- A case study.
- A self or peer-assessed piece of work.
- Any item submitted and judged to be appropriate by the student.

    — the structure of the portfolio;

    — a list of sample items;

    — the number of items required (Biggs suggest that four is the maximum in a semester-length unit);

    — the size of items and the overall portfolio;

    — any required items.

Decide how the portfolio will be assessed. It is suggested that global assessment of the whole portfolio is preferred to analytical marking to ensure that the broader purposes of students reporting and evaluating their learning are preserved and not broken down into discrete elements.

ASSESSING STUDENTS WITH A DISABILITY

Institutions have implemented many policies and practices to assist students with a disability. Unfortunately, consideration of their special needs is not always extended to the assessment of their learning. It is good practice for staff in departments to review and share alternative assessment arrangements on a regular basis as such arrangement are likely to be specific to both the kind of disability and to the nature of the discipline.

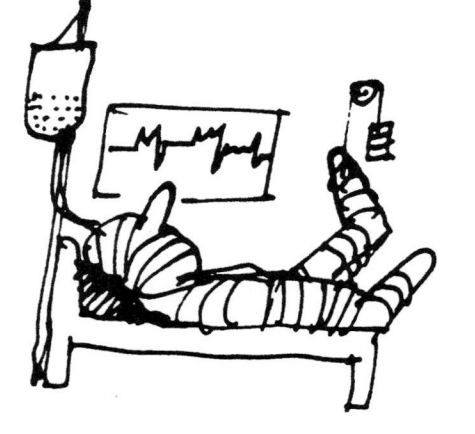

You are not expected to lower academic standards to accommodate these students but rather to provide them with a reasonable and fair opportunity to demonstrate their learning. Thus, you may need to make adjustments to assessment tasks once you understand how the particular disability affects performance. Space does not allow us to go into all the possible options here, but the following suggestions listed in Figure 8.20 for specific disabilities will give your students more equal opportunity in your course. Common strategies will be to simply follow good assessment practices we have described elsewhere and to be flexible in your insistence on assignment deadlines and in the time allowed in formal examinations.

ASSESSING STUDENTS AS GROUPS

With the increasing use of group and team-based learning, such as in problem-based learning, there is the related challenge of assessing the outcomes of group learning in ways that are fair to individuals but which recognise the particular dynamics and realities of such learning. More detailed descriptions of this assessment approach are given in Miller et al. and in Brown and Glasner, but the following ideas will be helpful when assessing group assignments.

FIGURE 8.20.
ASSESSMENT SUPPORT STRATEGIES

DISABILITY	ASSESSMENT – SUPPORT STRATEGY
MOBILITY DISABILITY	ALLOW STUDENTS A COMBINATION OF WRITTEN AND ORAL EXAMINATION BUT ALLOW STUDENTS TO PLAN THEIR ORAL ANSWERS EITHER VERBALLY OR IN WRITING TO ASSIST IN THEIR SPOKEN PRESENTATION
MEDICAL DISABILITY	ALLOW TAKE AWAY EXAMINATION TO ENABLE STUDENTS TO BE IN A COMFORTABLE ENVIRONMENT WHERE SUPPORT SYSTEMS ARE AVAILABLE
PSYCHIATRIC OR PSYCHOLOGICAL DISABILITY	POSTPONE ASSESSMENTS WHEN THE DISABILITY ENTERS AN ACTIVE PHASE; REDUCE ANXIETIES BY PERMITTING TEST TO BE UNDERTAKEN PRIVATELY AWAY FROM PERCEIVED THREATS OR DISTRACTIONS

Preparatory matters are important. Remember to keep group size down (greater than six members is too large); help students to work as effective group members; form groups randomly and change membership at least each semester; and ensure all students understand the assessment mechanisms you will use to encourage the diligent and forewarn the lazy.

Marking group submissions can be a way of assessing more students but taking up less time on your part. When allocating marks, the following strategies will be helpful:

- Give all members of a group the same mark where it was an objective to learn that group effectiveness is the outcome of the contribution of all.
- Give the group a mark to distribute as they determine. For example, if the group report was given a mark of 60 per cent and there were 4 members, give the group 240 (4 x 60) to divide up. This will be best managed if you have forewarned the group and assisted them with written criteria at the onset as to how they will allocate marks. An alternative is to have members draw up a contract to undertake certain group responsibilities or components. Components may be marked separately, or students may be given the task of assessing contributions themselves.
- Enhance the reliability of this form of assessment by conducting short supplementary interviews with students (e.g. What was your contribution? How did you reach this conclusion?) and build project-related questions into any final examination.

USING TECHNOLOGY IN ASSESSMENT

Computer technologies can be used to support assessment and we suggest you explore the facilities that are likely to be available to you in your own institution. There are several ways in which technology can be used. These include:

- As a management tool to store, distribute and analyse data and materials. An assessment system should be integrated with larger systems for curriculum management such as processing of student data and delivery of course materials.

- As a tool in the assessment process such as for the marking and scoring of tests. Answers from objective-type tests can be read by an optical mark reader and results processed by computer. However, more elaborate tools are now available to assess students work directly. Software can be purchased that enables you to prepare, present and score tests and assignments. You should check to see if your institution has a licence for some of these software products.

- As a resource for student learning and assessment. Basically, this involves students using technology to prepare and present work for assessment. Some simple examples include students preparing essays using a word processor or completing tasks using a spreadsheet application and submitting their work via e-mail. E-mail can also be used to provide a mechanism for the all-important feedback process from the teacher or from other students if collaborative group work or peer assessment is being used.

We recognise that information technology and telecommunications can be helpful and positive tools or resources for assessment. But we also have serious reservations about the way technology is being used as a tool in the assessment process. This is because the technology is so well suited for the administration and scoring of objective-type tests of the multiple-choice or true/false kind. We are seeing something of a resurgence of this kind of assessment in higher education with all of the well-known negative influences this may have on learning when items are poorly constructed or test only recall. All we can do here is urge caution, use good-quality test items, and to always ensure that students receive helpful feedback on their learning.

FEEDBACK TO STUDENTS

Major purposes of assessing student learning are to diagnose difficulties and to provide students with feedback. Several approaches to doing this have already been identified in this chapter and some of the methods described readily lend themselves to providing opportunities for feedback. To be specific:

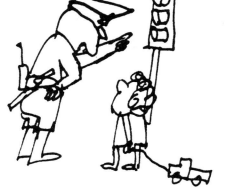

- use structured written feedback on essays;
- provide immediate feedback on technical, interpersonal, or oral skills as an outcome of direct observations, orals or practical assessments; and
- use self-assessment which includes feedback as part of the process.

Some guidelines for giving feedback include the following:

- keep the time short between what students do and the feedback;
- balance the positive with the negative;
- indicate how the student can improve in specific ways;
- encourage students to evaluate themselves and give feedback to each other; and
- make the criteria clear when setting work and relate feedback to the criteria.

REPORTING THE RESULTS OF ASSESSMENT

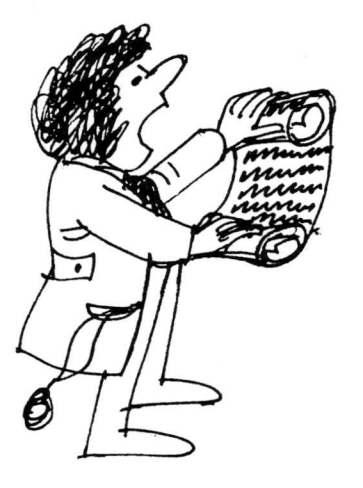

In many major examinations you will be required to report the results as a final mark or grade based on a number of different assessment methods. What usually happens is that marks from these different assessments are simply added or averaged and the final mark or grade awarded. Simple though this approach may be, it can introduce serious distortions. Factors contributing to this problem may be different distributions of marks in each subtest; varying numbers of questions; differing levels of difficulty; and a failure to appropriately weight each component.

The answer is to convert each raw subscore to a standardised score. This is not the place to do more than alert you to the need to do so and refer you to a text on educational measurement or to advise you to enlist the aid of an educational statistician, who can usually be found by contacting the teaching unit in your institution.

GUIDED READING

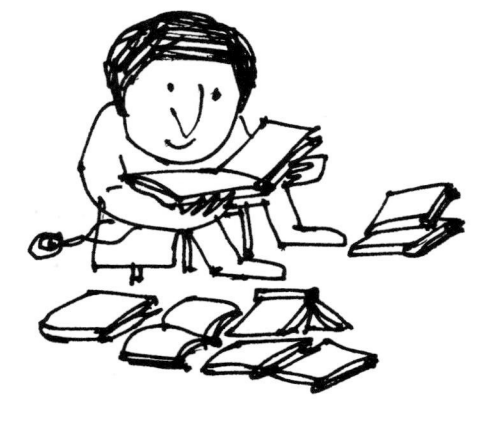

There are many useful general texts on educational measurement. An example is N. Gronlund's and R. Linn's **Measurement and Evaluation in Teaching**, Merril Press, Bellevue, Washington, 2000. Most will have useful discussions of broad assessment considerations such as objectives, planning, reliability, validity and scoring, and also will provide a wide range of examples of test items that you could use as models for your own tests.

Assessment Matters in Higher Education by S. Brown and A. Glasner, SRHE and Open University Press, Buckingham, 1999 is another general overview text that we recommend because of the many examples relevant to higher education.

We can also recommend *Student Assessment in Higher Education* by A. Miller, B. Imrie and K. Cox, Kogan Page, London, 1998, *Assessing Student Learning in Higher Education* by G. Brown and others, Routledge, London, 1997 and Chapter 9 in *Teaching for Quality Learning at University* by J. Biggs, SRHE and Open University Press, Buckingham, 1999.

A useful adjunct to this chapter is *Assessing Clinical Competence at the Undergraduate Level* by D. Newble; *ASME Medical Education Booklet No 25*, ASME, Edinburgh, 2000.

Books and articles referred to in this chapter

D. Boud (1995). *Enhancing Learning Through Self Assessment*, Kogan Page, London.

S. Case and D. Swanson (1996). *Constructing Written Test Questions for the Basic and Clinical Sciences*, 2nd edition, National Board of Medical Examiners, Philadelphia. It is available online at: http://www.nbme.org/new.version/item/htm.)

R. Harden and F. Gleeson (1979). Assessment of medical competence using an objective structured clinical examination (OSCE) *Medical Education*, 13, 41-54.

J. Norcini (1999). Standards and reliability: when rules of thumb don't apply. *Academic Medicine*, 74, 1088-1090.

9: PREPARING LEARNING AND TEACHING MATERIALS AND USING TECHNOLOGY

INTRODUCTION

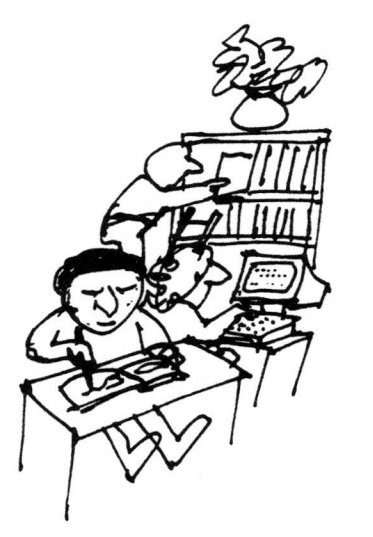

This chapter has proved to be challenging to write. The reasons for this are not hard to understand – there is now such rapid development in the application of computers and information communication technologies in higher education that much of what is said today is out-of-date tomorrow! On the other hand, it is fair to judge that as one looks around our campuses, for much of the time most teaching can still be described as 'traditional' with student groups of varying sizes meeting with a teacher for a set period of instruction. While we would not wish to see all of traditional teaching preserved for its own sake, it is nevertheless the case that it is in these settings, as well as in more contemporary approaches to learning and teaching, that we find a continuing need for assistance with such fundamental issues as using an overhead projector properly and preparing well-designed handouts.

We have addressed the challenge in three ways. First, from the previous edition we have updated material on some of the more basic technologies and retained a focus in this chapter on materials and technologies rather than on approaches to teaching. Teaching approaches are presented elsewhere in this book, for example, in the chapters on small groups and problem-based learning. Second, we have provided introductory ideas on using information technologies, and finally, we have distilled some principles of good practice that we believe apply to the use of all technologies and that provide a benchmark against which to evaluate what you are doing with your students.

BASIC PRINCIPLES IN PREPARING LEARNING AND TEACHING MATERIALS

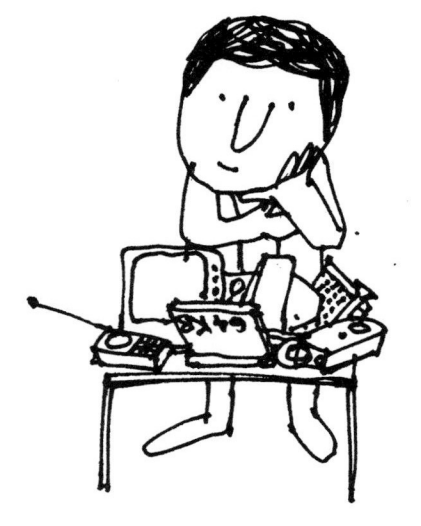

In your teaching career you will use quite a wide range of teaching materials and technologies. How you might produce and use them is the focus of this chapter. The fundamental criterion for judging the effectiveness of your teaching material is its audibility and/or visibility. If that seems too obvious to warrant mention, have a look at some of the materials used by others: overheads and slides with excessive amounts of tiny detail that cannot be read on the screen; complicated Web pages that look like art shows and take for ever to load on your computer; and faded handouts that cannot be read. Exaggeration? It does happen! When it does, it seriously interferes with the effectiveness of learning. Attention to the way in which the material is produced and how it is used in teaching will eliminate many of these problems.

Whether you are preparing a simple handout or multi-media materials, there are some basic principles that can be incorporated into your design and preparation that will enhance the quality and effectiveness of the material.

Relevance

Materials should be relevant to the purpose for which they were created and to the students' level of understanding of the topic. Complex handouts distributed at the end of a lecture and never referred to by the teacher are classic offenders of this principle.

Linkage

An introduction is usually required to establish the purpose of the material and to link it with what it is reasonable to expect students to know already.

Simplicity

Simplicity in the use of language and design, the avoidance of needless qualifications and the use of suitable abstractions of complex situations can be positive aids to understanding. For example, a simple line diagram may be more helpful in an explanation than a full-colour photograph or a complicated computer graphic.

Emphasis

Emphatic 'signs' can be incorporated into all teaching materials to stress important ideas, to indicate a change in the development of an argument, or to identify new material. Examples of emphasis include: headings and underlining in print; the use of colour and movement in Web pages; and statements such as 'this is a major factor' or 'to summarise these issues' on a sound recording of a lecture.

Consistency in the use of pattern and style

Students acquire a 'feel' for the particular style you use to present material. Needless changing of style is only going to confuse them. In the increasingly corporatised world of modern education, many institutions have now adopted a house style. You should check for its application to the preparation of your teaching materials.

TYPES OF LEARNING AND TEACHING MATERIALS AND AIDS

With these principles in mind, the preparation and use of several common types of teaching materials and aids will now be described. These are:

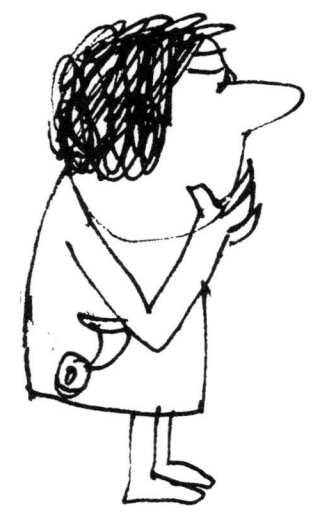

1 The overhead projector
2 The 35 mm slide projector
3 The video projector
4 The whiteboard and blackboard
5 Video and film
6 Printed materials
7 Material on the World Wide Web

This list is by no means exhaustive. In keeping with the general thrust of this book, the intention is to get you started and to help you develop some confidence in the basic aspects of your teaching work.

1. THE OVERHEAD PROJECTOR

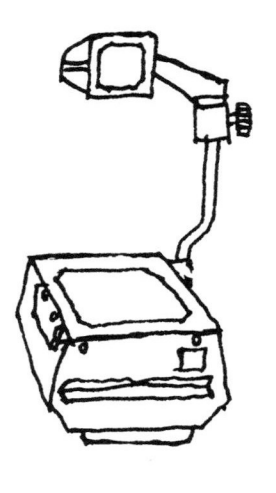

This valuable visual aid can project a wide range of transparency materials and silhouettes of opaque objects on to a screen positioned behind the teacher. Because it can project both written and diagrammatic information, it reduces your need to engage in detailed descriptions and increases the opportunities for discussion with students. It also allows you to indicate material on the transparency without turning your back to the audience, an advantage over using a slide projector or a whiteboard.

The full benefit of the overhead projector will not be realised in your teaching unless you give careful attention to three things: the preparation of the transparency, the way the projector is set up in a room or lecture theatre, and the way you actually use it. We shall now turn to a consideration of each of these matters.

Transparency preparation

Figure 9.1 shows what a transparency looks like. In its basic form, it consists of an acetate sheet mounted on to a cardboard frame. Additional sheets of acetate on the same frame are known as overlays. Overlays are particularly helpful to build up an idea as a presentation develops. Often, however, teachers dispense with the cardboard frame.

FIGURE 9.1.
EXAMPLE OF TRANSPARENCY

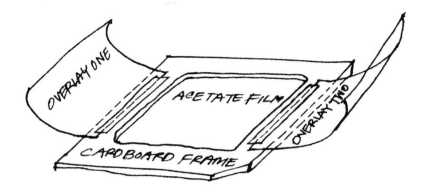

The following methods of making transparencies are available.

Felt pens: felt pens containing water-soluble or permanent ink are available for making transparencies. Information is printed or drawn directly on to an acetate sheet. A suggested procedure is to place a piece of ruled paper underneath the acetate as a guide and write on to the sheet. Another sheet of clean paper placed under your hand will prevent smudges from appearing on the acetate. Lettering should be no smaller than 5 mm in height and preferably larger. Use black, blue, brown or green pens for lettering, avoiding red, orange and yellow which are difficult to read at a distance.

Photocopying: plain-paper photocopiers will accept acetate sheets, enabling the production of transparencies at the touch of a button. It is essential that the type of transparency sheet selected is suitable for use with the copier and that the original material is large and clear. Lettering, for example, must be at least 5 mm in height. Avoid the temptation to make overheads directly from books or from typed materials. In general, transparencies made in this way will be invisible to most of the class and useless, unless students are each given an exact copy of the transparency as a handout. If you wish to use such material you should first make an enlargement.

Presentation packages: software presentation packages (such as PowerPoint) give you a means of producing master sheets for high quality transparencies. They also enable you to make and project transparencies electronically. If you are not already familiar with one of these packages, we recommend that you enrol in a short course to learn how to use it well. You will discover that making overheads is only the beginning! You will also be able to produce handouts, notes, and multi-media presentations incorporating pictures, movies and sound as well as text and diagrams of many kinds. Your finished work can be presented as slides and overheads using video projectors or standard equipment, via the Internet, and on desktop computers. The time required to learn to use a package will pay handsome dividends and open up a range of possibilities for you to make high quality materials.

When making overhead transparencies using this kind of software, remember the principle of simplicity – avoid the risk of overpowering your students with complex typefaces, distracting background designs and inappropriate colours. Learn some simple concepts of presentation design as well as how to master the technology.

Other uses of the overhead projector

There are other, less orthodox ways in which you can use the overhead projector. Silhouettes of cardboard cut-outs or solid objects can be projected on to the screen. These may be co-ordinated with a prepared transparency. Transparent or translucent materials such as liquids in test tubes or biological specimens mounted on, or contained in, clear containers can also be prepared.

The guidelines listed in Figure 9.2 should be kept in mind when preparing an overhead transparency.

FIGURE 9.2.
GUIDELINES FOR MAKING AN
EFFECTIVE OVERHEAD
TRANSPARENCY

Guidelines

★ Limit each transparency to one main idea.
  Several simple transparencies are preferable to a
  complicated one.

★ Reduce tabulated data to essential or to rounded
  figures. A single graph or diagram is often
  preferable.

★ Lettering on overheads should be at least 5 mm, or
  at least 24 points in height, and preferably much
  larger. Titles and headings should be in the range
  36-48 points.

★ Learn to use one of the commercially available
  presentation packages as a tool for making overheads.

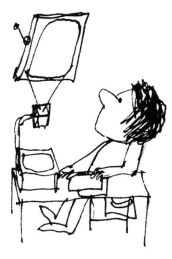

Setting up and using the overhead projector

In some situations you will have flexibility in setting up the
projector and screen. It is usual to place the projector so
that it is adjacent to the lectern or table from which you are
working. Ensure that the projected image is square on the
screen and free from angular and colour distortions.
Angular distortions in the vertical axis can sometimes be
overcome by tilting the top of the screen forward. Colour
distortions, such as red or blue in the corners of the
projected image, can usually be remedied by making an
adjustment to the lamp. A control for this is often inside the
projector. It is important to turn the electricity off at the
power point before the adjustment is attempted.

Whenever a projector is moved, or before a presentation
is commenced, the focus and position of the image must be
checked. Once this is done, it is usually unnecessary to look
at the screen again, particularly if you use a pen or pointer
directly on the transparency. This enables you to maintain
eye contact with students. If you wish to mask out part of the
transparency, place a sheet of paper between the film and
the glass stage of the projector. The weight of the
transparency should prevent the paper from moving or
falling away.

Remember to allow students plenty of time to read what
you have projected. Many teachers find this difficult to do.
One way is to read carefully the transparency to yourself
word for word. As well, make sure that anything you have
to say complements the transparency. Do not expect

students to listen to you and to look at something on the screen that is only vaguely related to what is being said. It is advisable to have the lamp on only when a transparency is being used in your teaching otherwise the projected image or the large area of white light will distract the students' attention.

2. THE 35 MM SLIDE PROJECTOR

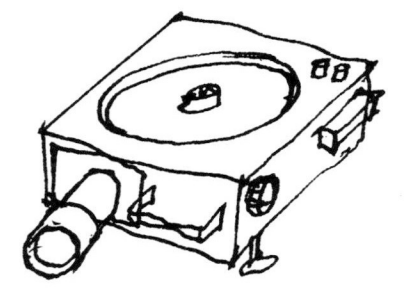

Much of what has been said about the overhead projector applies to slide projection. However, you will recognize that there are important differences between the two and that one of these is that full-colour images can be used in slides. This may be an advantage but with some material it may also be a disadvantage, unless the students' level of understanding is sufficient to enable them to see what is relevant and pertinent in the material you are using. Slide interpretation can be aided by including in the photograph an appropriate reference point or a scale.

Slide preparation

The major error in slide making is to assume that legibility in one medium, such as a table in a book or a journal, ensures slide legibility. Slides made from printed materials frequently contain too much detail and fine line work to enable them to be projected satisfactorily. This means that you may need to have artwork redrawn and new lettering added. Check any slides in your possession for legibility. A useful rule of thumb is that a slide which can be read without a magnifier is generally satisfactory. A better method is to go with a colleague to a large lecture theatre, project your slides and check to see if all details are legible and understandable at the rear of the auditorium.

When making slides, avoid the temptation to put all the details into the slide. If it is important for students to have all the details, provide these in a handout so that they can refer to it and keep it for reference. This ensures that they have accurate information on hand.

Photographers will advise you on the different processes available to produce your slides. These processes will usually include simple black-on-white slides, colour slides and diazo slides (white against blue, green or red backgrounds, the blue being preferred for clarity). Your institution may also be able to help you produce computer-generated colour slides of high quality. Another attractive and inexpensive way to prepare slides is to obtain negatives (white-on-black) and colour the white sections in by hand using coloured marking pens. The possibility exists for using separate colours to highlight different points on the slide. Whatever you choose, try to achieve a degree of consistency by sticking to one type of slide. Guidelines for the preparation of effective slides are given in Figure 9.3.

FIGURE 9.3.
GUIDELINES FOR MAKING
EFFECTIVE SLIDES

Guidelines

➡ Limit each slide to one main idea.

➡ Reduce tabulated data to essential or to rounded figures. Simple graphs and diagrams are to be preferred.

➡ When making new slides use a template with an aspect ratio of 3:2. An outline for typing of about 140 mm x 95 mm or 230 mm x 150 mm for artwork is suitable.

Setting up and using the slide projector

Slide projection equipment is normally part of the standard fixtures in a lecture theatre or seminar room so the question of setting up does not usually arise. If it does, locate the projector and screen with care to give the best view to students and so that it is convenient for you to operate the projector and room lights with a minimum of fuss. A remote control device will be an invaluable aid.

Slide projection

Before loading your slides into a carousel, carefully plan the sequence of their use. If your teaching is to be interspersed with slides, consider using black slides to separate your material and to avoid having to keep turning the projector on and off or leaving an inappropriate slide on view. Black slides are simply pieces of opaque film mounted in a slide frame to block off light to the screen and can be easily made from exposed film. If you plan to use the same slide on more than one occasion during a

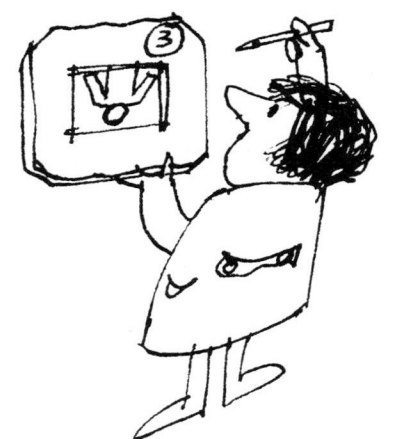

presentation, arrange to have duplicates made to save you and your students the agony of having to search back and forth through a slide series.

It is essential to have your slides marked or 'spotted' for projection (see Figure 9.4). As a check, the slides should be upside down and emulsion side (i.e. the dull side) towards the screen. When showing your slides, it is rarely necessary to turn off all the lights. Remember that students may wish to take notes and so you should plan to leave some lights on or to dim the main lights. Further advice on using slides is given in Chapter 4 on presenting a paper at a conference.

FIGURE 9.4.
PROCEDURE FOR 'SPOTTING' SLIDES

Procedure

1 Place your slides on a light box (an overhead projector is ideal for this) so that the image is the same way up as it is to appear on the screen.

2 Turn the slide upside down.

3 Mark or number the slide in the top right-hand corner.

---

3. THE VIDEO PROJECTOR

This exciting device enables you to project a variety of materials from a computer onto a screen for large and small group viewing. These materials include videos, broadcast television, slides and overheads, multi-media presentations, computer output, and Internet displays. When it is professionally set-up, supported, and used, the video projector is an outstanding presentation tool. Regrettably, this is often not the case. In our view, the current situation with video projectors is one that must be approached with caution as it is a good example of the embarrassing immaturity of much educational technology. If you doubt this judgement, have a close look at the systems currently in use with cords and cables everywhere, the need for backup computers, incompatible software and systems, the risk of system crashes, and so on! It is probably unwise to rely on a video projector system unless you are very familiar with its use and even then be well prepared with back-up resources.

Preparation

Your preparation involves four distinct matters: preparation of your material, familiarisation with the use of the equipment, arrangement of the teaching room, and production of back-up resources.

The preparation of your material is covered elsewhere in this chapter, keeping in mind the simple rule that whatever material is used, it must be clearly visible and audible! We urge you to consider producing back-up resources and alternative teaching strategies in case something should go wrong. For example, if you intend to be teaching in an unfamiliar environment or place, take overhead transparencies.

Equipment preparation can be broken down into understanding and preparing of the computer hardware and software, the operation of the projector itself, and the way the projector and computer are linked together. These are matters that need to be addressed well before any use of equipment is undertaken before an audience. To believe you can sort matters out in front of an audience is to invite disaster. If you cannot get tuition or expert assistance, take time to study equipment manuals and try out the procedures well in advance of any teaching or presentation commitment.

As with all projection equipment, you will need to give consideration to siting your video projector in relation to the room. In particular, review the position and focus of images on the screen, the level of illumination in the area of the screen, and the position of equipment and where you will be speaking in relation to the audience.

4. THE WHITEBOARD AND BLACKBOARD

The whiteboard is a ubiquitous presentation tool found in many meeting rooms as well as in classrooms these days.

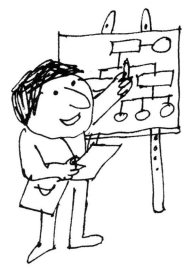

The principles of board use and preparation are outlined below. Do take care to use the correct pens with a whiteboard as some can ruin its surface. Also take care when cleaning a whiteboard. A dry cloth is often adequate but sometimes you may need to use water, detergent or perhaps methylated spirits. Never use an abrasive cleaner as it will scratch the surface and do irreparable damage to the board.

The colour of the pens you use is important. Black, dark blue and green are best. Avoid yellow, red and light colours, as these can be difficult to read from a distance.

The blackboard (which these days may be green) is still a commonly used visual aid and the one that you may use frequently, unless you rely exclusively on the overhead or video projector.

Few teachers give much thought to the material that they put on the board or to the way they use it. This is a pity. The results of the work are often ugly and indecipherable. Well-planned and well-used board work is a delight to see and is a valuable ally in presenting information accurately and clearly to your students.

Preparation

It is important to think ahead about your use of the board and make suitable notations in your teaching notes. Plan your use of the board by dividing the available space into a number of sections. Each section is then used for a specific purpose such as references, diagrams, a summary of the structure of the lecture, and so on.

Using a board

Some guidelines for using a board are given in Figure 9.5.

5. VIDEO AND FILM

Video gives you the opportunity to experiment with novel approaches to producing teaching materials, particularly now that relatively cheap cameras are available as well as presentation packages which enable you to integrate your video in a multi-media presentation. However, you should also become familiar with the range of suitable commercially or Web-based materials before embarking on a career as a producer. You will find that several subject areas are well catered for in this regard.

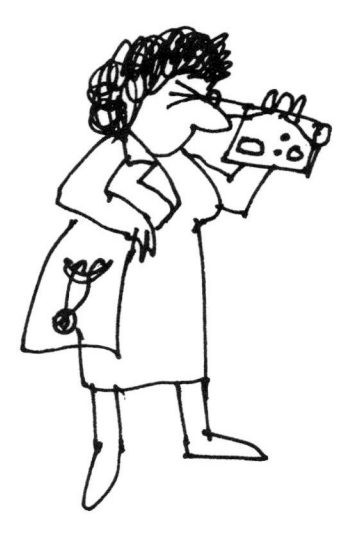

FIGURE 9.5.
GUIDELINES FOR USING BOARDS

GUIDELINES

- Start your teaching with a clean board. Clean your board when you have finished, both as a courtesy to the next class and also to reduce the likelihood of staining the board's surface.

- Try to avoid talking and writing on the board at the same time. When speaking, look at the students, not at the board.

- Face the board squarely and move across the board when writing. This will assist in writing horizontally.

- Stand aside when writing or drawing is completed to enable students to see the board.

- Concise information in skeleton note form is preferred to a 'newspaper' effect.

- Underline headings and important or unfamiliar words to give visual emphasis.

- Always give students a chance to copy down the information you have taken time to put on the board (if it is intended that they should have a copy).

- Use colours with discretion. Yellow and white are suitable colours for most written work on a blackboard, black and dark blue are best on white boards. Avoid using red, dark blue and green chalk sparingly as they are difficult to see and difficult to erase and avoid red and orange on white boards as they are relatively more difficult to read.

Although the uses of video and film are similar, video does offer you several additional advantages such as ease of production and relative cheapness. These have tended to make this medium more popular and flexible than film.

Using video and film in teaching

As with many teaching aids their uses are restricted only by your imagination and by the resources at your disposal. Some of the potential uses of video and film are described below.

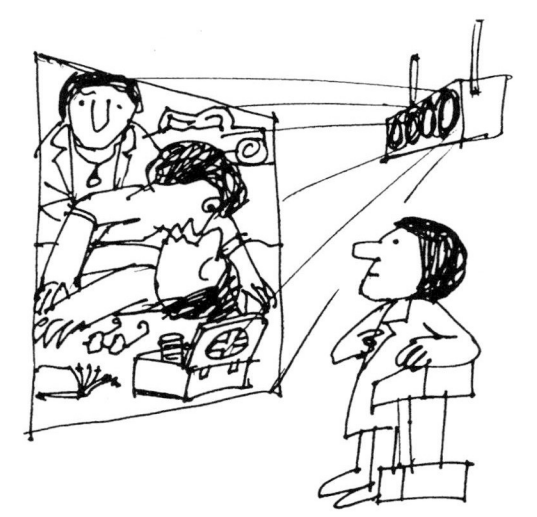

As introductory material: video and film can be used at the start of a course of study to stimulate interest, to provide an overview and to form a basis for further learning and teaching. For example, a film on the effects of cigarette smoking could be used as an introduction for a study of lung cancer.

As a major source of information: a constant flow of new ideas, techniques and procedures are a fact of life in most disciplines. Video and film can be used to disseminate this new information to your students or to professional meetings with which you may be involved. A further advantage of these media is that they can provide the viewer with vicarious experience where this might be difficult or dangerous to obtain at first hand.

As a means of modelling: this use is similar to the previous use, but you may find it helpful to produce material which demonstrates a technique or procedure in a clear step-by-step manner that students can watch and emulate at their own pace. An example might be a demonstration of how to conduct a clinical interview with a patient.

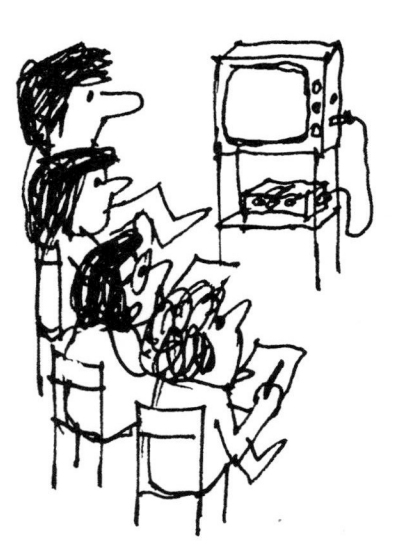

As a stimulus for discussion: short open-ended sections of video or film can be made to stimulate discussion among students. These are known as 'trigger films'. Students respond to the material as it is presented and both the stimulus and their responses are then discussed. This we have found to be valuable for starting discussion about attitudes dealing with emotional situations. Sometimes it is possible to locate suitable stimulus material in old films that would otherwise have no use.

As a means of distribution and relay: carefully placed video-cameras can be used to distribute pictures to a separate viewing room or even to relay them to remote locations. An obvious example of this is their use in operating theatres to enable a large number of students to witness an operation.

As an information storage system: video has a role to play in storing information for later teaching or for research use. For example, a recording can be made (with permission) by a student of a patient interview which can be reviewed later with a tutor at a convenient time and place.

As a means of assembling visual and audio information: in the past, video and film have been used to assemble a variety of information into one 'package'. Film clips, stills, models, interviews, recorded sounds and graphics can be recorded, assembled and edited to make a teaching programme. Today, presentation packages provide an accessible tool to achieve the same kind of outcome.

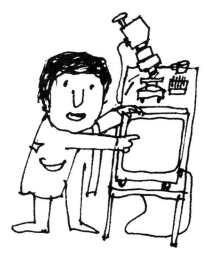

As a magnification medium: many teachers find that video is a handy tool to 'blow-up' the action or to display pictures of a demonstration. These can, of course, be recorded if needed for subsequent use.

These examples of video and film use are by no means exhaustive nor are they mutually exclusive in their application. For example, in teaching anatomy, video is used to magnify materials, to distribute and display this in a large laboratory (thus ensuring that all students are seeing the same thing) and sometimes to record the information as a resource for independent learning.

It is becoming less likely that you will be called on to produce videos for use in teaching. However, if you do, we recommend that you review the guidelines on making educational videos contained in earlier editions of this book.

6. PRINTED MATERIAL

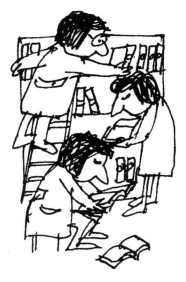

Books, journals, handouts and study guides carry a very large part of the instructional burden in teaching and will continue to do so in both paper and electronic media. Yet, often, surprisingly little thought is given by university teachers to the design and use of these important materials.

Design

We strongly recommend Hartley's book as a reference to have beside you. Care needs to be taken in designing and preparing printed materials. Over-organisation of the text does not help the reader and may actually interfere with learning. You will find it helpful to standardise on layouts. For example, in a paper-based system, you may wish to institute a system of coloured papers for different kinds of material you prepare for students (e.g. white for lecture notes, green for bibliographies, yellow for exercises). The basic principles for layout and design of printed materials are outlined in Figure 9.6.

FIGURE 9.6.
GUIDELINES FOR DESIGN OF
PRINTED MATERIALS

Guidelines

Incorporating the following can enhance learning from printed materials:

- An introduction to relate the new material to the past experience of the student.
- A summary of the major ideas or arguments presented.
- The use of major and minor headings.
- Space between paragraphs and sections to relieve the impact of too much print.
- Simplicity in expression.
- Appropriately labelled illustrations, tables and graphs (a series of diagrams building up to a complete concept may be more helpful than one detailed diagram).
- Questions and exercises within the text to stimulate thinking.

The variety of fonts available in personal computer software makes it necessary to select with care. Have a look at the typographical layouts in better-quality newspapers and journals for ideas that you can put into practice.

Using printed material

Handouts can serve a number of useful purposes in your teaching, but this medium is frequently misused because the material is often simply distributed to students and then quickly forgotten. Remember that you can produce handouts with the presentation software to support a formal lecture and that you can distribute them via the Internet.

Handouts can be used by students as a note-taking guide to a lecture. Supplementary information, or perhaps a copy of a paper you think is important, can also be given in a handout.

How you use the handout in your teaching is a crucial matter. We suggest that your students' attention be directed to the handout by discussing a particular definition, reading through a brief list of points with students, or asking them to fill in some part of it with additional information. If your students have to use the handout in the teaching session, it is likely that they will remember it and not simply file it away to be forgotten.

Prescribed reading

Prescribed reading of textbooks and journals is another matter that warrants your careful attention. Some teachers swamp their students with lists of books and articles to be read and give little thought to how students might manage the task. If you want the students to undertake some reading, then consider the following points:

- What are students expected to achieve by undertaking the reading? (Make this purpose clearly known to the students.)
- How will the reading be followed up in subsequent teaching?
- Will the recommended reading be readily available in libraries, through bookshops, or on the Web?
- How can the reading be usefully organised? (Arrange the material in a logical fashion, indicate why an item has been listed and what is especially important about it.)

7. PUBLISHING MATERIAL ON THE WORLD WIDE WEB

Preparing and publishing your own material on the Web should not be too difficult a task, particularly if you can enlist the assistance of locally available expertise to get you through the main technical issues. If you cannot locate such direct assistance then we suggest you either visit your local bookshop or computer retailer for the most recent books and software on the topic or seek advice on a current Web site for on-line help.

As the 'Internet revolution' matures the tools you need are becoming simpler. At the time of writing, the following general directions were valid. All you will need is a computer with a connection to the Internet and a 'web browser', which is the software that allows you to navigate through the different sites on the Web.

The basic steps are:

- Prepare your material. Your word processor may have an automatic 'Save As . . . HTML' option under the File menu. If so, your work is now ready for placement on the Web. This is the easiest option for preparing your material. The drawbacks are that some formatting may be lost and some punctuation marks altered. You also miss out on using more versatile Web building tools that can offer greater options (images, page colour, links to other sites etc) and thereby influence the way you may wish to present your material.

- Another option for preparing your work for the Web is to access free on-line Web page builders available from sites such as Geocities (www.geocities.com) or The Globe (www.theglobe.com). Or you can purchase one of several entry-level web page design software packages such as Adobe Pagemill or Netscape Composer. These packages come with helpful paper-based guides and they will enable you to save your work in a format that is ready for publication on the Web.

- Once your material is ready for the Web you need to place it on a 'server', that is a computer that is dedicated to the task of allowing viewers to access your page from anywhere, at anytime. For teaching uses, server space will usually be available from your institution. Space is also available through ISPs (Internet Service Providers). Alternatively, you may wish to take advantage of free server space offered through many sites on the Web. You will pay a price, though, usually in the form of a banner advertisement that displays when someone views your page!

You're done! Details on all the points above are available on the Web itself. If you are using or plan to use Netscape Composer, Netscape provides an excellent step-by-step guide (<http://home.mcom.com/browsers/createsites/index.html>).

As with all teaching preparation, you need a clear idea of what you are trying to achieve and for whom you are preparing the material. Assuming the material is for your students you could provide them with a diversity of resources to assist them with their learning, such as links to helpful learning resources, assignments and general feedback, reading material, examples of exemplary student work, and so on. Alternatively, you may be planning to teach interactively via the World Wide Web. In both of these cases, we urge you to review the currently available literature on the topic, some of which is identified in the Guided Reading section.

USING TECHNOLOGY IN LEARNING AND TEACHING

New technologies are having a significant impact on learning and teaching in higher education and will continue to do so. As we have already seen in this chapter and elsewhere in the book, computer and communication technologies can enhance a wide range of traditional teaching activities from the production and distribution of materials to the ways in which learners and teachers interact with each other. But these are examples of the ways in which technology replicates traditional teaching.

It is now clear that the forces of change are combining to move us to different ways of learning and teaching where we will see more of the following developments:

- students becoming more active and independent in their learning
- students working collaboratively with each other rather than competitively
- teachers becoming more designers and managers of learning resources, and guides for their students rather than dispensers and controllers of information
- rapidly changing curriculum content reflecting freedom to access a diverse range of ever-expanding resources for learning
- more effective assessment with a growing emphasis on assessment for learning.

How can you respond to these new and challenging demands and where can you learn more? Of course we hope that the material in this book will assist you with the basics of learning, teaching and assessment issues. But how can you learn more about the technologies (if these are new to you) or how can you keep abreast of developments? These matters are well beyond the scope of this book and so we hope the following Guided Reading will be helpful.

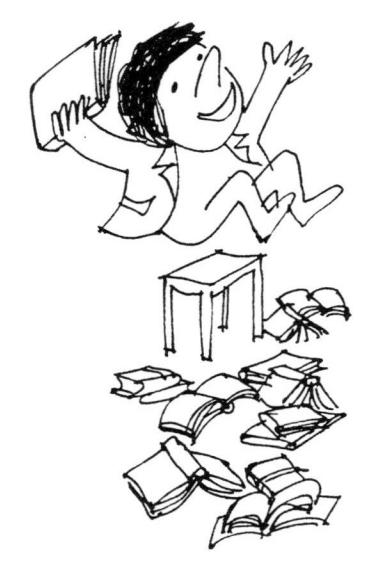

GUIDED READING

For those new to technology, and in particular the technologies applied in higher education, we recommend two complementary books. The first is by A. Warren et al., *Technology in Teaching and Learning: An Introductory Guide*, Kogan Page, 1998. The second is by P. Maier et al., *Using Technology in Teaching and Learning*, Kogan Page, 1999. The first book takes the reader through the fundamentals of using computers and the second book explores ways in which computers can be used to support the teaching of large groups, to deliver learning resources to students, and for communication between students.

If you want to go further, and explore more of using the Internet in your teaching, we suggest I. Forsyth, *Teaching and Learning Materials and the Internet*, Kogan Page, 2000.

To maintain your currency in the uses of technology beyond the material in these books we urge you to monitor the literature in books, journals and especially in the electronic resources of the kind available on the World Wide Web.

There is rapidly growing number of books, as well as resources on the Web, that can assist you with some of the educational issues of using technology in education. We suggest the following three books:

- A. Inglis, P. Ling and V. Joosten, *Delivering Digitally: Managing the Transition to the Knowledge Media*. Kogan Page, London, 1999.
- R. Phillips, *The Developer's Handbook to Interactive Multimedia, A Practical Guide for Educational Applications*. Kogan Page, 1997.
- D. Brooks, *Web Teaching*. Plenum Publishing Corp, New York and London, 1997.

If you are concerned to evaluate materials and educational technologies we suggest M. Tessmer, *Planning and Conducting Formative Evaluations*. Kogan Page, London, 1993. This is an interesting mixture of useful guidance on planning evaluations, evaluating materials, and the whole notion of formative evaluation. Hartley's book (see below) is also helpful on evaluating materials.

Books referred to in this chapter:

J. Hartley, *Designing Instructional Text* (3rd edition), Kogan Page, London, 1994, is highly recommended for preparing text-based materials (books, manuals, handouts, computer-generated or stored text). We used Hartley when preparing this book.

10:   THE EVALUATION OF
LEARNING AND TEACHING

INTRODUCTION

There is an increasing demand that university teachers provide evidence of their teaching effectiveness for purposes of appointment, tenure and promotion. As a result we have included this new chapter which we hope will help you in three important ways.

- Provide you with information and resources that will assist you to evaluate your teaching and the learning of your students.
- Guide you in ways that will assist you to make good use of the information you create through your evaluative activities.
- Arm you with ideas on how to improve the practice of evaluation in your institution.

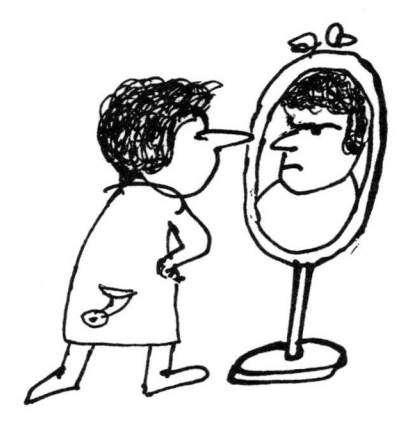

The third is especially important and is often overlooked. In our experience, as many difficulties in evaluation are created by the implementation of poor policies and practices as by the processes of collecting and presenting evaluative information. One poor practice is an obsession with quantification. This has led to an over-emphasis on those things that can be most easily counted, such as student ratings of a teacher's behaviour, and an under-emphasis on those areas of academic work less easy to quantify such as learning processes or advising students.

There is another important factor here as well. Just as the ways we go about assessing our students will directly influence their learning behaviours, so too will the ways institutions evaluate their teachers drive teacher behaviour. For example, the strong emphasis on research in many universities is, in part, a direct consequence of the way we evaluate and reward this academic activity by promoting people on the basis of their research output and grant income generation. This may compete with activities required to perform teaching duties at a high level.

Before we address these matters in more detail, we want to outline the context in which we are presenting ideas to you and to clarify some important concepts.

THE CONTEXT OF EVALUATION

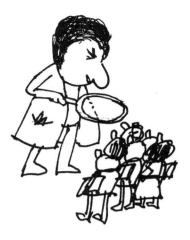

Evaluation and learning

Evaluation is an important part of the process of learning. It is to do with finding out from our students about the quality of their learning and obtaining information about the effectiveness of our teaching. How can we do this? We shall be suggesting some ideas about this after we have briefly reviewed another important side of evaluation – accountability.

Evaluation and accountability

One of the most dramatic shifts in higher education practice in the past decade has been the move towards accountability. By 'accountability' we mean a demand to provide clear evidence of what is being done in higher education and of the outcomes of learning and teaching. This evidence is then used in a variety of ways, one of which of major interest to you is decisions about academic promotions and contracts.

At the national level, governments are generally under pressure to account for the way public funds are used and so exert a corresponding pressure on institutions to improve their effectiveness. Owners and trustees exert similar pressures in the non-government sector of higher education. Institutions are thus required to gather data about learning and teaching and present it as evidence for their claims of effectiveness and quality.

Institutions, in turn, have exerted accountability demands onto faculties, teaching departments and individuals. They commonly require that courses be evaluated on a regular basis and that teachers evaluate their teaching and use the information obtained for both the improvement of teaching and of courses.

Evaluation: some definitions and principles

Evaluation is a process of obtaining information for judgement and decision making about programmes, courses and teachers. Assessment, a term which is sometimes used interchangeably with evaluation, is about obtaining information for judgement and decision making about students and their learning. However, the results of an assessment of student learning is a very important part of evaluation.

We are sure you will be familiar with some of the ways commonly used to gather information – questionnaires and interviews for teaching evaluations, and assignments and examinations to assess student learning. Strategies for judgement and decision-making are less well-developed, however, and we will look at these later in the chapter.

You should keep in mind two broad intentions behind evaluation. The first is *formative evaluation*. This is intended to assist in change, development and improvement of teaching. The second is *summative evaluation*. This is used to make decisions such as whether to promote or re-appoint a teacher.

Whatever the intentions of an evaluation, you will find it useful to keep in mind that there are several sources of evaluative information and methods you can use to get this information. These matters are summarised in Figure 10.1 and Figure 10.2

FIGURE 10.1.
SOURCES OF INFORMATION FOR AN EVALUATION

What are some sources for an evaluation of learning and teaching?	What are some examples of valid information they can give you?
People sources	
Students	Course implementation; teaching behaviors
Academic colleagues	Contribution to the administration of teaching
Graduates	Relationship of courses to work
Observers	Descriptions of what is occurring
Professional associations	Comparative data against some agreed standard
Self	Satisfaction; allocation of resources (time)
Administrators, Departmental Heads, Deans	Administration, commitment, innovation
Employers	Satisfaction with graduate skills
Material sources	
Course materials	Teaching plans and philosophies, administration
Products of student learning and assessment results	Learning outcomes
Files/records	Administrative matters, student data

Different methods are available to gather information from these sources. For example, if you are particularly interested in the students' experience, you may decide to use several different methods including diaries, questionnaires and focus groups. Some of these methods are listed below in Figure 10.2.

FIGURE 10.2.
METHODS AND TECHNIQUES FOR AN EVALUATION

What are some methods of gathering information?	In what ways can these methods be used?
Questionnaires	Surveys of student, graduate, employer opinion
Interviews	In-depth exploration of issues
Students' diaries/work records/logs	Learning activities, processes and reaction
Discussion (focus group, panel)	Identification of issues in teaching or courses
Comments (both solicited and unsolicited)	Student reaction to a broad range of issues
Observation of student/teacher behavior	Learning processes; teaching behavior
'Unobtrusive' observation (e.g. noting the extent of students' use of recommended books)	Students' learning activities
Feedback sections on homepages attached to an e-mail address	Almost all areas of teaching and other facilities
Results of student work	Learning
Personally gathered information (teaching portfolio)	Documenting and describing teaching

Space does not allow us to explore all of these sources and methods, which of course can be used in a wide range of combinations. For more help, we recommend you consult someone in your institution's teaching unit or review the references provided at the end of the chapter.

However, in deciding among the options in the table, you need to be aware that two fundamental characteristics of evaluation are validity and reliability. Other important characteristics are the practicality of an evaluation and, of course, its acceptability to all those involved.

Validity refers to the truthfulness and appropriateness of information provided as evidence of learning and teaching. For example, high levels of student achievement may not be a valid indicator of teaching competence because of the problem of identifying the relative contribution of teacher, student effort, library resources, students' peers, and so on. On the other hand it is a valid indicator of learning. Students can provide valid feedback on the availability of resources and teacher behavior, for example, because they observe and experience these things as part of their course.

191

Reliability refers to the extent to which information provided is dependable and consistent. For example, information about a teacher based on the results of just one student survey will not be as reliable as information derived from several surveys conducted over several years and from a representative range of classes taught. The reliability of an evaluation may also be enhanced if different, but valid methods, are used in combination.

Now, armed with this background knowledge, how might you go about evaluating your teaching? There is one important preliminary matter to consider – planning.

Planning evaluation as part of your teaching

Among the things you need to think about are the following:

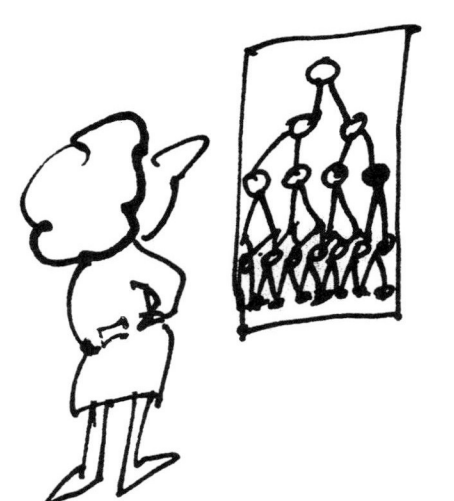

- Determine what are your institution's formal requirements for evaluation. For example, is there a requirement that you should gather student feedback on a regular basis for curriculum development or for promotion or tenure?
- Make contact with the staff of your teaching unit who will at least be able to advise you if not provide direct evaluation services to you.
- Draw up your own plan of evaluation. As we have already suggested, evaluation is an important element of good teaching and so it is something you should be doing all the time.

Matters you will need to consider in your plan are how and when you will evaluate your teaching, how you will evaluate student learning and what you will do with the information you gather. You must have some plan to use the information in ways to improve or develop learning and your teaching otherwise there is little point in doing it at all. One way of using information will be to incorporate it into an on-going record of your work known as a Teaching Portfolio. We explain this below. Another important way of using information is to ensure you give your students feedback on the outcomes of your evaluations and what it is planned to do with the results. Practical ways in which you can communicate this kind of information are through your personal or departmental Web page, or by posting information on the student notice board.

THE EVALUATION OF LEARNING AND TEACHING

Evaluating learning

As with all evaluation, the process of evaluating learning consists of two major elements: gathering information and then making judgements based on that information. What sources of information are there about learning? The reliability of your evaluation of student learning will be enhanced by your judicious use of more than one valid measure of learning. So, what is available? The first, and major source of information about student learning, will be the results of your programme of student assessment – the examination results; assignments and projects; reports; clinical notes, and other products; and observations of student learning.

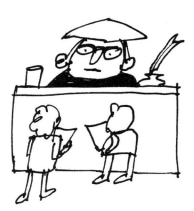

In our experience a great deal of useful information from students is overlooked. For example, it is necessary to go beyond the scores and grades from tests, and to ask questions about learning, for example:

- What are common errors – and how can I address these in my teaching?
- In what areas have students shown particular strengths, weaknesses, interests and why might this be so?
- What misconceptions are evident in students' work – and how can I address these in my teaching?
- What levels of intellectual achievement are revealed in students' work: for example, do they simply appear to rote learn or is there evidence of analysis and critical thinking?
- What feedback will I give students and how will I do this?

This process of questioning and thinking about one's teaching is a fertile way of developing an understanding of student learning so that you can modify teaching and provide additional assistance to students if this is indicated.

A second way of evaluating learning is through well-designed and administered evaluations of teaching. There is a considerable body of research evidence that shows this to be a valid approach provided that the questions ask about factors related to learning and not something else!

Information about how students are progressing in achieving the goals of your teaching can be found in questionnaire items such as:

● I have understood the concepts presented in the subject.
● I have a positive attitude to this subject.
● My ability to work independently has been increased.
● My ability to think critically/solve problems/perform clinical tasks/etc. has increased.

Apart from formal questionnaire surveys, you will find that evaluation by brainstorming an issue with your students (such as 'are the course objectives being achieved?') can be a very powerful learning experience for all involved!

The third way you can obtain information about the processes of learning is by using tools such as CATs (Classroom Assessment Techniques); two examples of which we have already mentioned in Chapter 2.

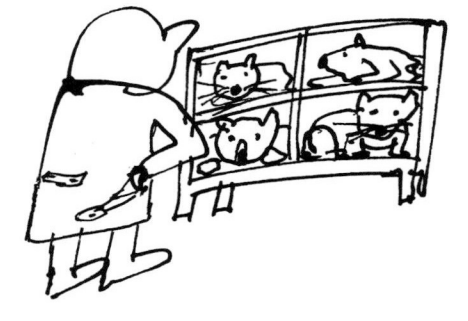

Another CAT has been developed to help teachers evaluate student reaction to exams and tests and to improve these as effective learning and assessment devices. Called the Exam Evaluation, the procedure for using this evaluation tool is:

● Focus on a type of test you are going to use more than once.
● Develop questions that you would like to ask of students. You might also consider asking students what questions they would like to be asked.
● Choose the questions and decide whether you will ask these at the end of a test or as part of a follow-up evaluation. Examples of questions are 'Did you learn more from one type of test than another?' 'What is it about the test that accounts for this?' 'Was the test a fair assessment of your learning?' 'What are the reasons for your response?'

In their book *Classroom Assessment Techniques*, Angelo and Cross describe 50 different CATs so an exploration of these is well worth the effort. CATs not only give you useful information about learning, but research has shown how they can have positive instructional benefits such as increasing students' perceptions of the quality of their learning and the level of activity by stimulating class participation. One of the most important elements of good teaching is feedback and CATs can help in this. Of course, it is essential you give your students feedback on the outcomes of these exercises too! Remember one of our key principles is that 'Reliable and valid assessment of learning and giving helpful feedback on students' work is a distinguishing characteristic of good teaching.'

Evaluating learning in these ways will yield a rich variety of information. But it may be lacking in one important respect and that is, it may not indicate ways in which you can improve. To do that, you have to ask your students (and maybe your colleagues too). There are a number of ways you can do this that range from a frank discussion with an individual student, or a group, to sophisticated student rating systems.

Evaluating your teaching

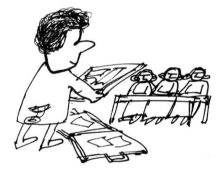

As we have seen from Figure 10.2, questionnaires are only one way you can gather information about your teaching. Depending on what you wish to evaluate and why, we think you will find it necessary to use more than one technique. For example, several of our colleagues use focus groups where issues are explored in depth with small groups. They also arrange to visit each other's classes for observation and feedback. Increasingly, some are also using e-mailed questions and feedback from students as a means of evaluation.

Examples of evaluation tools are given in various parts of this book. We also suggest, if you do not have ready access to an evaluation service on your campus, that you consult one of the many books on the subject. Centra gives examples of several questionnaires in his book and we think you will find these helpful.

If you decide to use questionnaires we suggest giving careful consideration to the following:

- That the evaluation questions asked of students accurately reflect the learning and teaching they have experienced; that is, they are 'valid'.
- That students are able to answer questions based on their direct experience of teaching (for example, a first

year student will generally not be in a position to judge whether a teacher's subject knowledge is up-to-date, whereas a graduate student or colleague may well be able to make such a judgement).

● That when an individual is being evaluated for summative purposes that only responses to questions about matters that the individual can reasonably be held accountable for are used and reported on.

In recent years there has been considerable innovation in medical teaching and the evolution of methods, such as problem-based learning and computer-assisted instruction, where teams of teachers are more commonly responsible for development and implementation. At the same time there has been an expansion of teaching at the graduate level where individual supervision of research projects is common. These different approaches to teaching demand different approaches to evaluation and the points we have made above apply to these as well. If you find yourself teaching in one or more of these situations we think you need to be fully aware of the general issues we have presented here and to also seek help and guidance from the more specialised literature (some of which we comment on in the Guided Reading section) or from staff in your teaching unit.

Recommendations for using evaluations for developmental purposes (formative evaluation)

The outcomes of all your evaluations should be included in your Teaching Portfolio. An important part of any portfolio is a section in which you complete a critical self-review, or 'reflection', about your teaching. We say more about this below.

As well as having a plan of action, the other major recommendation we can make is to discuss the outcomes of an evaluation with someone, perhaps an adviser or consultant on teaching, or a trusted colleague or mentor. In addition, a frank discussion with your students will yield two positive benefits. First, it gives them feedback on the outcomes of the evaluation and about your plan to act on the information they have given you. Secondly, you will be able to clarify some areas and seek suggestions from them for changes.

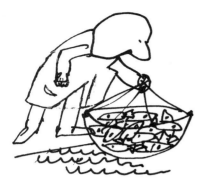

Recommendations for using evaluations for administrative purposes (summative evaluation)

In this rather longer part we summarise some of the currently available ideas from research about using evaluations for administrative purposes such as promotion or tenure. Because you will find that there is on-going debate and dispute about some of these recommendations, we have provided some references so that you can review the findings and more detailed reasoning behind them.

- It is more appropriate to document and describe your achievements in teaching and to relate these to your specified duties and expectations than it is to pursue some quantitative criterion, such as a 'magic number' derived from evaluative data (e.g. a score of 6 on a 7-point scale). Several sources of valid evaluative information are preferred over any single source. For example, a portfolio approach which combines peer evaluation, student evaluation, and appropriate evidence from other sources is recommended (Magin, 1998).

- If questionnaires are used, short rating forms with fewer global items are recommended rather than forms containing a large number of heterogeneous items. Examples of global items should relate to a teacher's responsibilities – 'the stated aims were achieved', 'accessible to students', and 'feedback provided promptly' or an overall rating of effectiveness rather than to stylistic questions ('I liked the presentation techniques' or 'enthusiastic') (Scriven, 1981; Magin, 1998).

- Whatever kinds of statistical scores are used in a report on teaching, that only broad categories of final judgement be made (such as 'outstanding', 'adequate', and 'unacceptable'; or 'promote' and 'do not promote') (McKeachie, 1997).

- The circumstances under which evaluations are collected and analysed are appropriate and rigorously applied. Standardised procedures should be used for legal and ethical reasons (d'Apollonia and Abrami, 1997).

- Evaluations should be collected before final examinations (d'Apollonia and Abrami, 1997).

- You should avoid comparing teachers by using numerical means or medians. Comparisons of ratings from different groups, even within a specific discipline, is a very dubious exercise because of a myriad of variables such as between-class differences among students; teacher's gender; different goals, learning and teaching methods, and assessment arrangements; different course content; and varying degrees of difficulty. Just as important as the mean or median, is the spread of scores – the standard deviation – which raises issues of how much variation in perception of experience exists within groups. Comparisons are not necessary for personnel decision making. What is necessary is evidence to allocate the teacher to one of two or three broad categories, such as 'promote' or 'do not promote' and this can be achieved by looking at the overall distribution of student ratings on key questions such as teacher effectiveness (McKeachie, 1997).

A key observation made in McKeachie's paper (p.1218) can be a guiding principle in using student evaluations for summative purposes. He declares: ". . . the basic problem is not with the ratings but rather with the lack of sophistication of those using them for personnel purposes."

BRINGING IT ALL TOGETHER: A FRAMEWORK FOR THE EVALUATION OF YOUR TEACHING

By now you will be aware of the complexity of evaluation and we hope that the following framework will help you think about the ways in which you evaluate your teaching and also other aspects of your academic work. For example, our focus is on the documentation necessary to assist in a summative evaluation. However, this focus can incorporate both formative evaluation of teaching and the evaluation of learning because the process of thoughtful documentation is likely to stimulate thinking about your practices which may, in turn, lead to improvements.

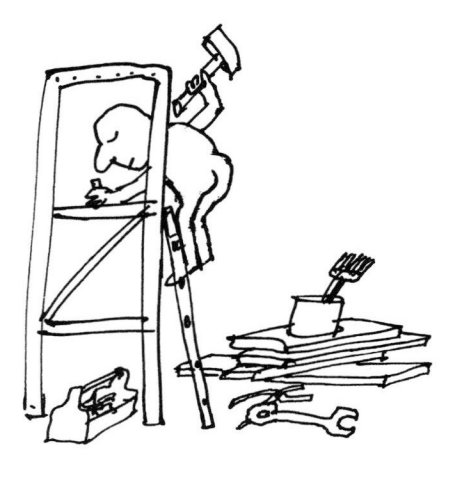

In a major publication on evaluation by Glassick et al., 1997, a broad framework is proposed which is intended to apply to all forms of academic scholarship, including teaching. Applied to teaching and learning, the main elements of the framework are:

★ establishing standards of teaching as scholarly work
★ documenting teaching
★ ensuring a trustworthy system of evaluation.

Establishing standards

Teaching evaluation can be guided by the following qualitative standards. You will recognise most of these as they reflect the qualities of good teaching we keep reminding you about!

1 Clear goals
2 Adequate preparation
3 Appropriate methods
4 Significant results
5 Effective presentation
6 Seeking feedback

1. Clear goals

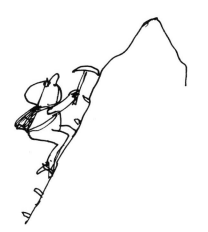

Having clear goals is one of the elements of the organisation of effective teaching identified by the research, but having clear goals is of little value if they cannot, realistically, be met. Consider the following:

● Have you stated the goals of your teaching in terms of expected learning outcomes?
● Have you defined goals that are clear, realistic and achievable?

2. Adequate preparation

Preparation involves the identification and bringing together of resources and materials to support teaching. The following questions may help you here:

● Do you demonstrate an understanding of existing scholarship in your field?
● Do you bring the necessary skills and understanding about learning and teaching to your work as a teacher?
● Do you obtain and organise the resources necessary to achieve your goals?

3. Appropriate methods

Methods and procedures appropriate to the goals and your context have to be chosen, applied effectively, and modified and adapted as teaching proceeds. Methods make a great difference in teaching, from the methods used to organise and present a syllabus, to learning and teaching methods, and the assessment arrangements. The following questions are relevant here:

- Do you use methods appropriate to the goals?
- Do you apply these methods effectively?
- Do you modify your methods in response to changing circumstances and feedback?

4. Significant results

Teaching will ultimately be judged by its results as well as the quality and integrity of its processes. We often ask about learning outcomes in our questionnaires to students: whether the teacher stimulated their interest, whether their ability to work independently has been increased, and the extent of their understanding. The significance of the outcomes of teaching might be judged by asking question like:

- ★ Did your students achieve your stated goals?
- ★ Does your scholarship in teaching make a difference to your students and to your field of work?
- ★ Does your work open up new areas for development or enquiry?

5. Effective presentation

The importance of presentation in teaching, whether it is presentation in a traditional lecture setting or the presentation of learning materials using an electronic technology, is of major significance. Teaching scholarship should also lead to presentation to colleagues, through publication and conferences, as well as presentation to students. The following questions are relevant here:

- Do you use presentation methods appropriate to your goals and teaching context?
- Do you use appropriate forums to present your teaching scholarship?
- Do you present with appropriate clarity and integrity?

6. Seeking feedback

The final standard involves the teacher's continuing learning about his or her work by actively seeking out feedback from others so that the whole process of teaching can be monitored and improved. Ask yourself:

- Do you regularly evaluate your own work?
- Do you bring to this evaluation a broad range of evidence?
- Do you critically integrate evaluation, reflect on it, and use it to improve the quality of your teaching?

Documenting teaching: the Teaching Portfolio

The second part of the framework is documenting your teaching. The purpose of documentation is to provide the evidence that can be used to judge the extent to which the standards have been achieved. Our purpose here is to focus on how you might record your academic achievements. A valuable tool in working towards this purpose is the teaching portfolio or teaching dossier.

Your portfolio might have three main parts:

- A statement of responsibilities defining what you were required to do, or had hoped to accomplish. This is the basis against which your work will be judged.
- A statement of your philosophy of teaching and learning, preferably in relation to your institution's goals and plans. This might also include a very brief biographical note outlining the breadth and depth of your scholarly work as a teacher.
- The summarised evidence of your achievements and effectiveness as a teacher. Figure 10.3 gives an extensive list of items that might be appropriate. This summarised evidence can be organised using the standards described above.

There are several reasons why we advocate the preparation and maintenance of a portfolio. These reasons are:

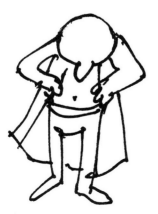

- **Self-evaluation**: the summary you prepare provides an invaluable record of your teaching which assists you to reflect on your teaching over a particular period (say a semester or year) and to make improvements should these be necessary.

- **Evidence for new appointments, tenure, annual review or promotion**: institutional appointments and promotions committees increasingly demand evidence of teaching accomplishments to assist them in their decision making. This reflects a worldwide emphasis on better quality teaching. So it is very wise to have maintained a portfolio for at least the past two or three years. A portfolio will also be very useful in your annual review.

- **Evidence in cases where your teaching is challenged**: in these days of increasing accountability and staff appraisal there may be occasions where the quality of your work is challenged. Documentary evidence maintained by you in your portfolio may prove invaluable in defending your case.

- **Fostering discussion and review of teaching**: keeping a portfolio and encouraging others to do so will help to create an environment where discussion of teaching becomes the norm rather than an unusual practice in your department.

Do remember that a teaching portfolio is a summary of your major teaching activities and accomplishments; it is an important adjunct to your curriculum vitae (CV). It is not intended that it include all the material listed in Figure 10.3. Accordingly, you should initially be comprehensive in your collection of information for your portfolio and then summarise the material when it is to be used for some external audience.

Creating, assembling and using your portfolio

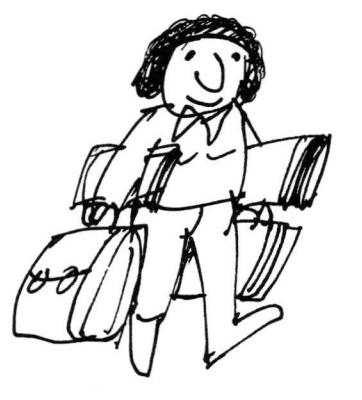

The most important things to remember are to keep evidence of your teaching activities and to file away a copy of relevant materials, letters received, articles published, evaluations conducted, and so on, and that your portfolio is a *summary*. The evidence is the basis from which your portfolio is constructed and the source from which any statements you make in your portfolio can be verified. It is suggested that your portfolio might end up being between six and twelve pages long.

To compile your portfolio we recommend the following steps:

- Clarify the purposes to which the portfolio will be put and choose appropriate criteria to describe and evaluate your teaching.
- Keep files of back-up material to follow the structure used in the portfolio. Remember, these materials are not part of the portfolio, but are evidence if required.
- Prepare brief statements of explanation against each of the criteria selected. You should also add your own brief evaluation of the item and the steps you have taken to modify your teaching in light of (say) feedback received.
- Incorporate the portfolio into your CV.
- Finally, remember to constantly review your portfolio and keep it up to date. It is surprising how easy it is to forget the diverse teaching activities we undertake and the feedback we receive. Remember too that your portfolio is an important tool for learning about your teaching. Use it for this purpose also!

Ensuring a trustworthy system of evaluation

The final part of the framework for an evaluation system is ensuring that the system in place is 'trustworthy'. We cannot go into much detail about this here, but the following quotation from *Scholarship Assessed* summarizes what we have in mind:

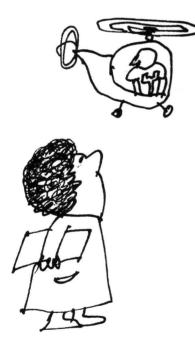

". . . successful evaluation would be a process with clear goals for institutional and individual performance and adequate preparation for evaluators and candidates. Appropriate methods would be used and significant results would advance the institution and individual towards their goals. The process would be effectively presented and discussed as openly as possible in public forums. Finally, reflective critique would keep evaluation flexible and open to improvement over time." (p.51).

We do not expect that you will be able to change your institution's policies and practices overnight. But, by talking about the characteristics of good evaluation with the right people, you will have an influence upon bringing about useful improvements for the advancement of learning and teaching.

FIGURE 10.3. POSSIBLE CONTENTS FOR A TEACHING PORTFOLIO

THE PRODUCTS OF GOOD TEACHING

1. Students' scores on teacher-made or standardised tests, possibly before and after a course has been taken as evidence of learning.

2. Student laboratory workbooks and other kinds of workbooks or logs.

3. Student essays, creative work, and project or field-work reports.

4. Publications by students on course-related work.

5. A record of your students who select and succeed in advanced courses of study in the field.

6. A record of your students who elect another course with you.

7. Evidence of effective supervision of Honours, Masters or PhD theses.

8. Setting up or running a successful internship or staff development programme.

9. Documentary evidence of the effect of courses on student career choice.

10. Documentary evidence of your help given to students in securing employment.

11. Evidence of help given to colleagues on teaching improvement.

MATERIALS FROM ONESELF
Descriptive material on current and recent teaching responsibilities and practices

12. List of course titles and numbers, unit values or credits, enrolment statistics with brief elaboration.

13. List of course materials prepared for students.

14. Information on your availability to students.

15. Report on the identification of student difficulties and encouragement of student participation in courses or programmes.

16. Description of how materials and resources were used in teaching (e.g. libraries, Internet, etc.).

17. Steps taken to emphasize the interrelatedness and relevance of different kinds of learning.

Description of steps taken to evaluate and improve one's teaching

18. Maintaining a record of the changes resulting from self-evaluation.

19. Reading journals on improving teaching and attempting to implement acquired ideas.

20. Reviewing new teaching materials for possible application.

21. Exchanging course materials with a colleague from another institution.

22. Conducting research on one's own teaching or course.

23. Becoming involved in an association or society concerned with the improvement of teaching and learning.

24. Attempting teaching innovations and evaluating their effectiveness.

25. Using general support services such as the Education Resources Information Centre (ERIC) in improving one's teaching.

26. Participating in seminars, workshops and professional meetings intended to improve teaching.

27. Participating in course or curriculum reviews.

28. Pursuing a line of research that contributes directly to teaching.

29. Preparing a textbook or other teaching materials.

30. Editing or contributing to a professional journal on teaching one's subject.

INFORMATION FROM OTHERS
Students:

31. Student course and teaching evaluation data which suggest improvements or produce an overall rating of effectiveness or satisfaction.

32. Written comments from a student committee to evaluate courses and provide feedback.

33. Unstructured (and possibly unsolicited) written evaluations by students, including written comments on exams and letters received after a course has been completed.

34. Documented reports of satisfaction with out-of-class contacts.

35. Interview data collected from students after completion of a course.

36. Honours received from students, such as being elected 'teacher of the year'.

Colleagues:

37. Statements from colleagues who have observed teaching either as members of a teaching team or as independent observers of a particular course, or who teach other sections of the same course.

38. Written comments from those who teach courses for which a particular course is a prerequisite.

39. Evaluation of contributions to course development and improvement.

40. Statements from colleagues from other institutions on such matters as how well students have been prepared for graduate studies.

41. Honours or recognition such as a distinguished teacher award or election to a committee on teaching.

42. Requests for advice or acknowledgment of advice received by a committee on teaching or similar body.

Other sources:

43. Statements about teaching achievements from administrators at one's own institution or from other institutions.

44. Alumni ratings or other graduate feedback.

45. Comments from parents of students.

46. Reports from employers of students (e.g. in a work-study or 'cooperative' programme).

47. Invitations to teach for outside agencies.

48. Invitations to contribute to the teaching literature.

49. Other kinds of invitations based on one's reputation as a teacher (for example, a media interview on a successful teaching innovation).

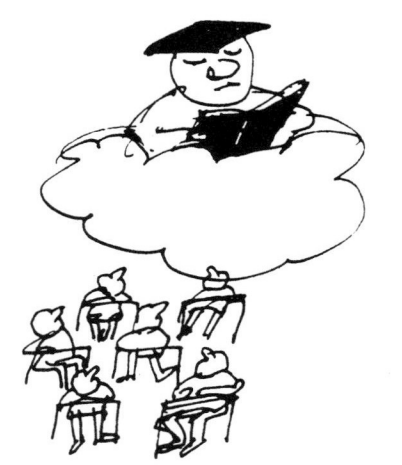

GUIDED READING

There is a wealth of material on evaluation and you may care to check your library's holdings for recent books and guides. A good overview of evaluation, the issues, methods, and resources is J. Centra, **Reflective Faculty Evaluation**, Jossey-Bass, San Franciso, 1993. This book also explores evaluating research and service and so complements **Scholarship Assessed** which is noted below.

On portfolios, the most straightforward advice is contained in the original Canadian work on this subject by B. Shore et al., **The Teaching Dossier, Guide to its Preparation and Use**, Canadian Association of University Teachers, 1991. Another useful introduction to portfolios, which also considers their relationship to scholarship, is **The Teaching Portfolio: Capturing the Scholarship of Teaching** by R. Edgerton, P. Hutchings and K. Quinlan, American Association for Higher Education, Washington, D.C., 1991.

If you are concerned to evaluate materials and educational technologies we suggest M. Tessmer, **Planning and Conducting Formative Evaluations**, Kogan Page, London, 1993. This is an interesting mixture of useful guidance on planning evaluations, evaluating materials, and the whole notion of formative evaluation. Hartley's book is also helpful on evaluating materials; **Designing Instructional Text**, Kogan Page, London, 1994.

Books and articles referred to in this chapter:

T. Angelo and K. Cross. **Classroom Assessment Techniques**, Jossey-Bass, San Francisco, 1993.

S. d'Apollonia and P. Abrami (1997). Navigating student ratings of instruction, **American Psychologist**, November, 1198-1208.

C. Glassick et al. **Scholarship Assessed, Evaluation of the Professoriate**, Jossey-Bass, San Francisco, 1997.

W. McKeachie (1997). Student ratings, the validity of use, **American Psychologist**, November, 1218-1225.

D. Magin (1998). Rewarding good teaching: A matter of demonstrated proficiency or documented achievement?

The International Journal of Academic Development, 3, 2, 124-135.

M. Scriven. Summative teacher evaluation. In J. Millman (ed), *Handbook of Teacher Evaluation*, pp. 244-271. Sage, Beverly Hills, 1981.

**APPENDIX:
WHERE TO FIND OUT MORE ABOUT
MEDICAL EDUCATION**

As a result of your involvement in teaching you may eventually wish to pursue in greater depth an interest in medical education. This section of the book will identify various resources which might be helpful.

BOOKS AND JOURNALS

We have already provided selected readings at the end of each chapter. There are some other texts which may be of more general interest and which cover a wider range than the selected readings.

On the principles of good teaching in higher education we suggest *Teaching for Quality Learning at University* by J. Biggs, SRHE and Open University Press, Buckingham, 1999 and *Learning to Teach in Higher Education* by P. Ramsden, Routledge, 1992.

An excellent introduction to the important concept of life long learning which covers a wide range of related teaching issues is *Lifelong Learning in Higher Education* by C. Knapper and A. Cropley, Kogan Page, London, 2000.

For those wishing to delve more deeply into aspects of medical education research there is now a major text entitled *An International Handbook for Research in Medical Education* by J. Norman, C. Van der Vleuten and D. Newble (eds), Kluwer Academic, Dordrecht, 2001.

Articles relating to medical education appear regularly in most of the major general medical journals. Many of these are now searchable on-line. There are also several journals specifically concerned with publishing research and review articles in the field of medical education.

Medical Education
This is the official journal of the Association for the Study of Medical Education (ASME), which is the organisation catering for individuals interested in medical education in the United Kingdom. It should be readily available in your medical school library.

The Association also produces an excellent series of booklets dealing with various aspects of medical education and has a series on medical education research. These are also published in the journal.

Academic Medicine (previously *The Journal of Medical Education*)

This is a publication of the Association of American Medical Colleges. As well as containing articles relating to teaching, this journal also deals with the broader issues of the organisation of medical education as it relates to the United States. It also publishes the *Proceedings of the Annual Conference on Research in Medical Education* which is the world's premier medical education research meeting.

Medical Teacher

This journal is now published in collaboration with the Association for Medical Education in Europe. In the past it has not been primarily a research journal. Rather, it has been a journal containing review articles and descriptions of educational activities by medical teachers from around the world. While this focus remains it is increasingly publishing quality research articles. It remains an excellent source of ideas and information.

Teaching and Learning in Medicine

An American medical education journal gaining a reputation as a major international journal. It often contains high quality research based reviews.

Advances in Health Sciences Education

A relatively new addition to the list of medical education journals. While published in Europe it has a prestigious international editorial board and is a source of high quality educational research and review articles.

World Health Organisation

The WHO has been very active for many years in the field of medical education. It frequently commissions experts to write review documents. A list of such publications should be available in your library. If not, you could write direct to Distribution and Sales, CH-1211 Geneva 27, Switzerland or search the WHO Website.

TRAINING OPPORTUNITIES

Many tertiary institutions have individuals or units whose job is to provide assistance to teachers. We would strongly recommend you make full use of these resources. Alternatively, you could elect to attend courses run by other organisations in your area or even overseas. The WHO supports regional teacher training centres which offer short courses for medical teachers and even degree courses in health personnel education.

Many universities now have medical education departments or units which run courses of various types and some have well-developed degree or fellowship programmes for local and overseas postgraduate students.

OVERSEAS TRAVEL

Generally speaking, people concerned with medical education are friendly and helpful. Should you be travelling, do not hesitate to write to any individual or institution you may wish to visit and observe at first hand educational activities or facilities which have interested you during your reading. If you come from a traditional medical school, you should attempt to visit one of the well known less conventional schools such as McMaster University in Canada; Maastricht University in the Netherlands; Ben Gurion University of the Negev, in Israel; or Newcastle University in Australia. Many other institutions are now experimenting with alternative curricula so opportunities to experience different ways of teaching medical students should be found reasonably close to your home institution.

ORGANISATIONS

As your interest in medical education grows you may wish to join an association or attend one of the national or international conferences which are held each year. The following is a list of some of the most well know English-speaking organisations which conduct major annual conferences.

Association for Medical Education in Europe (AMEE)

This is an umbrella organisation for national medical educational associations in Europe. It is also well supported by the WHO. In addition it provides a regular forum for the meeting of medical school deans from Europe and sometimes from other parts of the world.

Further information can be obtained from the Secretary, AMEE, Tay Park House, 484 Perth Road, Dundee, DD2 1LR, Scotland or on < www.dundee.ac.uk/MedEd/AMEE >

Association for the Study of Medical Education (ASME)

This is also a European organisation with a largely British membership but with a significant number of members from other countries. It caters for individuals with an interest in medical education and provides a forum for communication of ideas and information. It organises conferences and workshops and produces several publications including the well know ASME booklets series.

Further details can be obtained from the Secretary, ASME, 12 Queen Street, Edinburgh, EH1 1JE or on
< www.asme.org.uk >

Association of American Medical Colleges

This is another umbrella organisation covering medical schools in America. It holds an annual meeting and in conjunction with this is held the Research in Medical Education Conference. This meeting provides the major annual gathering of workers in the field of medical education in the United States and Canada.

Further information can be obtained from the AAMC, 2450 N Street N.W., Washington, DC 20037, USA or on
< www.aamc.org >

ANZAME: The Association for Health Professional Education

This is an association covering Australasia which holds an annual conference and also supports state and regional groups which meet on a regular basis. It publishes a journal *Focus on Health Professional Education*.

Further information can be obtained on
< www.anzame.unsw.edu.au >

International Ottawa Conferences on Medical Education

These are held every 2 years and have become the most popular international conferences on research and development in medical education. They take place in different countries each time. Information about future conferences can be found in the News Section of the journal *Medical Teacher*.

INDEX